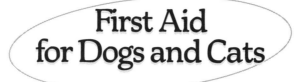

# First Aid for Dogs and Cats

Editor: Michael Ballantyne, Ginette Patenaude

**National Library of Canada cataloguing in publication**

Robinson, Chantale
    First Aid for Dogs and Cats
    Translation of: Premiers soins pour chiens et chats


    1. First aid for animals.    2. Pets - Wounds and injuries - Treatment.    3. Cats - Diseases -
    Prevention.    4. Dogs - Diseases - Prevention.    I. Title.

SF981.R62    2004            636.089'60252        C2004-940414-8

**EXCLUSIVE DISTRIBUTORS:**

• For Canada and
  the United States:
  MESSAGERIES ADP*
  955 Amherst St.
  Montréal, Québec
  H2L 3K4
  Tel.: (514) 523-1182
  Fax: (514) 939-0406
  * A subsidiary of Sogides Ltée

• For France and other countries:
  **INTERFORUM**
  Immeuble Paryseine, 3 Allée de la Seine
  94854 Ivry Cedex
  Tel.: 01 49 59 11 89/91
  Fax: 01 49 59 11 96
  **Orders:** Tel.: 02 38 32 71 00
            Fax: 02 38 32 71 28

• For Switzerland:
  **INTERFORUM SUISSE**
  P.O. Box 69 - 1701 Fribourg, Switzerland
  Tel.: (41-26) 460-80-60
  Fax: (41-26) 460-80-68
  Internet: www.havas.ch
  E-mail: office@havas.ch
  DISTRIBUTION: OLF SA
  Z.I. 3 Corminbœuf
  P.O. Box 1061
  CH-1701 FRIBOURG
  **Orders:** Tel.: (41-26) 467-53-33
            Fax: (41-26) 467-54-66

• For Belgium and Luxembourg:
  **INTERFORUM BENELUX**
  Boulevard de l'Europe 117
  B-1301 Wavre
  Tel.: (010) 42-03-20
  Fax: (010) 41-20-24
  http://www.vups.be
  Email: info@vups.be

For more information about our publications,
please visit our website: **www.edjour.com**
Other sites of interest: www.edhomme.com • www.edtypo.com
www.edvlb.com • www.edhexagone.com • www.edutilis.com

This book was originally published in French as
*Premiers soins pour chiens et chats,* © 2002,
Le Jour, éditeur ,la division of the Sogides Group

Legal deposit: third quarter 2004
Bibliothèque nationale du Québec

ISBN 2-8904-4739-1

The publisher gratefully acknowledges the support of the Société de développement des entreprises culturelles du Québec for its publishing program.

We gratefully acknowledge the support of the Canada Council for the Arts for its publishing program.

We acknowledge the financial support of the Government of Canada through the Book Publishing Industry Development Program (BPIDP) for our publishing activities.

Chantale Robinson

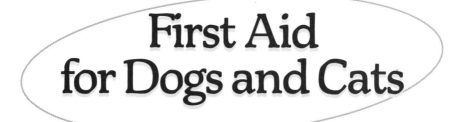

# First Aid for Dogs and Cats

*Translated by*
*My-Trang Nguyen*

le jour,
éditeur

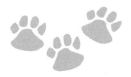

# INTRODUCTION

I chose to become an animal-health technician because I knew the profession would put me in daily contact with animals. It would also give me a chance to do what I loved, and do it with passion: providing pets with basic, indispensable health care.

My work often puts me in contact with injured pets, but it was a particular event that motivated me to write this book. I received a call for help one morning from a panic-stricken woman. She had run over her dog while backing up her car. "It's lying on the ground now," she said frantically, "and it's not moving or even breathing!" I tried to coach her about checking for the animal's vital signs and giving it artificial respiration, but she was sobbing and too upset to understand. How I wish I'd been there, by her side, so that I could have helped her more effectively.

I suggested that she come to the clinic immediately. As soon as she arrived, we rushed to examine the dog. But it was too late. All we could do was to pronounce the animal dead and do our best to console its owner. The poor woman blamed herself bitterly for her inability to save her dog.

I later realized that had she been familiar with first aid, she could have intervened on the spot and perhaps saved her pet's life. And that was how the idea for this book – *First Aid for Dogs and Cats* – came about.

Pets are a part of the family. They are also our responsibility and depend on us for their welfare. If we want to give them the best possible care, it is wise to learn techniques that can make the difference between life and death. I hope this book will offer the reader valuable help. Consult it frequently so that you can react confidently to emergency situations. This book is not intended to replace veterinary care, but it does include everything that a sensible pet-owner should know and do before heading for the veterinary clinic.

# ANATOMY OF A DOG

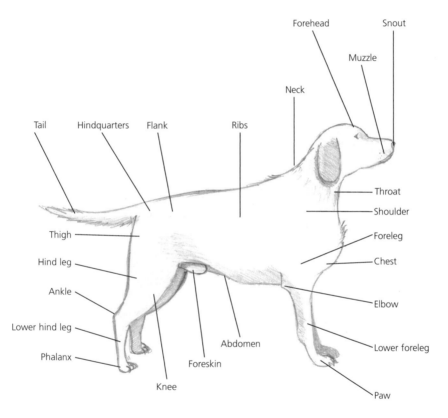

Forehead

Snout

Muzzle

Neck

Tail

Hindquarters

Flank

Ribs

Throat

Shoulder

Thigh

Foreleg

Hind leg

Chest

Ankle

Lower hind leg

Elbow

Phalanx

Abdomen

Lower foreleg

Foreskin

Knee

Paw

# ANATOMY OF A CAT

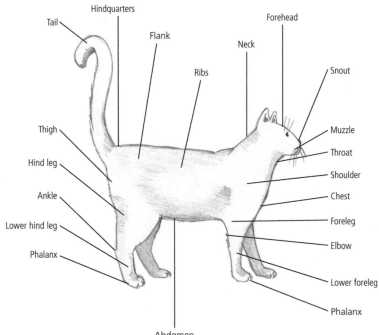

Tail

Hindquarters

Flank

Ribs

Forehead

Neck

Snout

Muzzle

Throat

Shoulder

Chest

Foreleg

Elbow

Lower foreleg

Phalanx

Thigh

Hind leg

Ankle

Lower hind leg

Phalanx

Abdomen

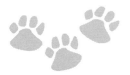

# Chapter 1
# VITAL SIGNS

The first step in assessing your pet's state of health is the ability to recognize what's normal, or abnormal, for each animal. Only then can you proceed to provide appropriate care, or decide to consult a vet, depending on the situation.

It's imperative, therefore, that you get to know your animal companion intimately. This will enable you to tell, at a glance, whether or not something is wrong. A dull coat or a lack of tonus and energy, for instance, may indicate a particular disorder. Moreover, feeling and touching the animal may reveal important clues about its health: you'll be able to detect potential problems more speedily, such as cuts, swellings, weight loss, etc. In addition, it's a good way of communicating with your pet, as you train it to get used to being touched by humans. The animal will become less fearful and more cooperative in emergency situations, especially when a vet is busy poking and prodding it. This is precisely why you should stroke your pet all over, from head to tail.

The vital signs, on the other hand, allow you to assess the animal's health with greater precision. They include body temperature, respiratory and heart rate, color of mucous membranes, blood circulation and degree of dehydration.

## Body Temperature

Warm-blooded animals must maintain a stable internal temperature in order to survive. It may fluctuate slightly, but any substantial change means that the animal suffers either from hyperthermia (fever, see page 118), or hypothermia (below average body temperature, see page 121). An animal's temperature is always taken rectally, using a thermometer.

You can't gauge your pet's health by merely checking the temperature of its snout. The animal may very well be running a temperature as high as 39.5°C (103°F) while the snout stays cold! Warm ears, on the other hand, may suggest a fever, while frozen ones point to hypothermia.

---

**NORMAL TEMPERATURES FOR CATS AND DOGS**
38°C – 39.1°C (100.5°F – 102.5°F)

---

### Taking your pet's rectal temperature

Use a mercury thermometer, or better still, a digital one, the latter being easier to read and more accurate.

Lubricate the thermometer with a petroleum (i.e. Vaseline) or lubricant gel.

Insert the thermometer about 2.5 cm (1 in.) inside the rectum (just under the tail), leaving it in place for three minutes or, if you use a digital thermometer, until it emits a beeping sound.

Read the temperature.

## Respiratory Rate

An animal's breathing may also reveal its state of health. A respiratory rate that is either too rapid or too slow signals discomfort, pain or a more serious problem. It's important that you become familiar with your pet's normal respiratory rate so as to detect any irregularities quickly. Also, observe it during the animal's various daily activities: when it's asleep, awake, at play, etc.

| NORMAL RESPIRATORY RATES | |
|---|---|
| **CATS** | **DOGS** |
| • Cats breathe 20 to 30 times a minute.<br>• When panting, a cat can breathe up to 300 times a minute.<br>• Cats normally pant in stressful situations (visits to the vet, when frightened, in hot weather). Such panting should last no longer than a few minutes at a time. If it persists and the cat doesn't revert to breathing normally, you should seek veterinary care ASAP (as soon as possible). | • A puppy breathes 15 to 40 times a minute.<br>• A full-grown dog breathes 10 to 30 times a minute.<br>• Miniature breeds breathe 15 to 40 times a minute.<br>• When panting, a dog can breathe up to 200 times a minute.<br>• Dogs normally pant in stressful situations (visits to the vet, when frightened, in hot weather). Such panting should last no longer than a few minutes at a time. If it persists and the dog doesn't revert to breathing normally, seek veterinary care ASAP. |

### Assessing your pet's respiratory rate

There are several ways:

- Keep an eye on the thoracic cage as the animal inhales and exhales, or place your hand on the animal's chest.
- Count the number of times the chest expands in 10 seconds and multiply it by 6; or in 15 seconds and multiply by 4. This will give you the animal's respiratory rate per minute.
- If you're not sure that your pet is breathing (for example, if it's unconscious), hold a cotton ball or a piece of tissue paper before its nostrils. If the cotton ball or tissue paper moves, the animal is breathing.
- A mirror can also be used to see if the pet is breathing. Hold it close to the nostrils to see if condensation forms.
- If the animal's abdomen, rather than its chest, expands while it is breathing, see a vet immediately.
- If the animal sounds as if it is gasping for air, or if its breathing is superficial, see a vet immediately.

## Heart Rate

It varies greatly depending on the animal's size and age: the smaller the animal, the faster the heartbeat. The following table gives a general breakdown of normal heart rates.

| NORMAL HEART RATES | |
|---|---|
| **CATS** | **DOGS** |
| • 110 to 130 heartbeats per minute. | • Puppies: 70 to 120 heartbeats per minute.<br>• Dogs: 70 to 180 beats per minute.<br>• Miniature breeds: 70 to 220 beats per minute. |

### Assessing your pet's heart rate

There are several ways of detecting an animal's heart rate. One is by pressing your ear against the animal's chest and listening to the heartbeat; another is by taking its pulse at various points on its body. The pulse refers to the rhythmic throbbing of a blood vessel as the heart contracts; it is obtained by lightly pressing your finger against an artery. If you can't take the pulse at a particular spot because of an injury, then select another.

### Listening to your pet's heartbeat

- Lie the animal on its right side. Flex its left foreleg so that the elbow is pressed up against its chest. You'll find that the heart is located just behind the elbow (toward the fifth rib). Heartbeats are perceptible at that point.
- Place your hand there and you'll feel the pulse. If not, press your ear against the animal's chest and listen. If the animal is obese, use a stethoscope, because the layer of fat can make the sound of the heartbeat difficult to detect.
- Once you've found the pulse, count the heartbeats in 10 seconds and multiply by 6, or in 15 seconds and multiply by 4, to obtain the heart rate per minute.

A regular heartbeat consists of a series of two beats separated by an interval: *TUM DUM, TUM DUM* (like a drum). If the rate sounds irregular to you, consider it an emergency and call the vet immediately.

### Taking the pulse

If for some reason you cannot detect a heartbeat by listening to the animal's chest, you can always take the animal's pulse at some position along an artery.

#### On the inner thigh (femoral pulse)

- Lie the animal on its side. If it won't cooperate, let the animal stand up.
- Slightly part its hind legs and place your hand along the inner thigh, in the groin area near the pelvis.
- To find the pulse, slide your index and middle fingers toward the middle of the leg, but not too far from the hip. A tendon runs through this spot and the femoral artery follows this tendon. Try to feel the pulse. Don't press too hard or you'll miss it.
- Calculate the femoral pulse the same way you count the heart rate.

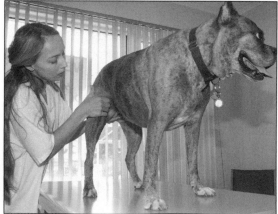

| FOREFEET | HIND FEET |
|---|---|
| 1. Select the middle plantar pad.<br>2. Place your index and middle fingers on the pad.<br>3. Find the pulse.<br>4. Calculate the pulse the same way you count the heart rate. | 1. Select the middle plantar pad.<br>2. Place your middle and index fingers on the pad.<br>3. Find the pulse.<br>4. Calculate the pulse the same way you count the heart rate. |

## Blood Circulation

There are clues that can tell you whether your pet's circulation is satisfactory, such as the color of the mucous membranes and the capillary refill time. These are especially useful if your pet suffers from internal bleeding or is in a state of shock.

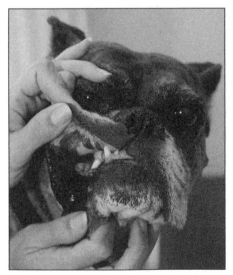

### Assessing the color of the mucous membranes

Pull the animal's lips open and examine the color of the mucous membranes and the gums.

Pink gums indicate good blood circulation and healthy tissue oxygenation. Any other color points to a disorder that must be treated immediately:

- Red or brick-colored gums suggest a slight state of shock.
- Pale pink or white gums are a sign of severe shock or bleeding.
- Yellowish gums suggest an unhealthy state.
- Bluish gums indicate that the dog is no longer breathing.

Certain breeds have naturally dark-colored mucus membranes and gums, which makes it more difficult to assess their condition. If this is the case, pull gently on the skin underneath the eyes, and examine the mucus membranes' color inside the eyelids.

### Assessing the capillary refill time

This test allows you to gauge your pet's circulation, and check for disorders such as anemia, insufficient blood flow or any state of shock.
- Lift the animal's lip and press a finger firmly against the gum above the canine.
- Remove your finger and see how long it takes for the gum to return to its original pink color.

The normal capillary refill time is one to two seconds. If it's less than one second, the pet is in a state of shock. If it's more than three seconds, the circulation is compromised. Call the vet immediately: it's an emergency.

## Dehydration

Dehydration, or tissue fluid loss, is a serious disorder that can quickly cause death. It is most often caused by vomiting and diarrhea. To find out whether or not your pet is dehydrated, grab the skin on its neck or back then release it. The skin should retract immediately, or after a second or two. If it hasn't done so after three seconds, your pet is dehydrated. Consult a vet at once.

On the other hand, the skin of an aging or emaciated animal loses its elasticity, making it harder to check for dehydration – it obviously takes longer to spring back to its normal position. If this is the case, check for other signs of dehydration: sunken eyes, for example, or dry and sticky gums (due to lack of saliva).

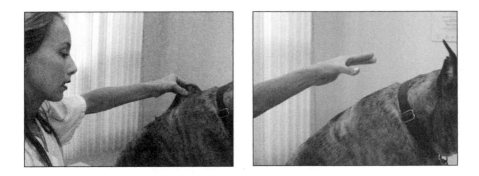

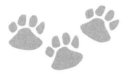

# Chapter 2
# EMERGENCY INTERVENTIONS

Before learning about the various pathological conditions and traumas that may affect your pet, and the first-aid care you need to administer in each case, it's important to master basic first-aid skills: how to approach an injured pet properly, for example, and handle it without aggravating its condition. You must also learn to recognize emergencies when they occur and to respond promptly. Finally, being familiar with such techniques as cardiopulmonary resuscitation (CPR) and the Heimlich maneuver may make the difference between life and death for your pet.

## Approaching, Immobilizing and Transporting an Injured Animal

In emergency situations, the first crucial step in first aid is the ability to understand animal language. Only then can you attempt to approach, immobilize and transport an injured animal.

## Body language

It's very important to understand an animal's body language when it is in distress. Before attempting to help it, make sure you proceed very cautiously, for even the gentlest of animal companions can bite if it's in pain or frightened. An aggressive dog grunts and snarls, bares its teeth and points the ears forward, signaling that it will bite if you come too close. A frightened dog simply grunts, its ears are pointed backward so that they lie flat against its head, its tail is tucked between its legs and the hair on its back erect. But beware: if threatened, it will bite.

A submissive dog doesn't normally attack but slumps to the ground, tail between legs, ears drooping, flank exposed. Sometimes, it will urinate. However, it, too, can bite if it's frightened or in pain.

A cat expresses fear explicitly: it falls to the ground, points its ears backward, then grunts, hisses or attacks by trying to scratch and bite.

## Approaching an animal in distress

- When you come face to face with an animal in distress, the first rule is to maintain a respectful distance and speak in a soft, gentle voice.
- Approach the animal slowly and gradually. If it shows signs of aggression, stay where you are and continue talking quietly so as to gain its confidence. If it still refuses to let you come near, don't insist on approaching.
- Avoid looking at an aggressive dog in the eye, because it will interpret that as provocation on your part.
- Call the nearest SPCA and warn people not to approach the animal until help arrives.

## Capturing and controlling an injured animal

A slightly injured animal tends to run away. So if you've managed to get close, try to immobilize the animal before providing first aid or taking it to a vet. As you apply the following techniques, stay within view of the animal so it won't be surprised or alarmed. Show the animal that you mean no harm.

- Use a nylon leash (never a chain) to make a running knot. Throw the knot around the animal's neck while keeping a discreet distance. Pull gently on the leash to tighten the knot[1]. In this way, you'll be able to prevent the animal from running off and avoid any risk of being bitten.
- If the animal's life is not in danger and it can walk, guide it to the car with the leash.
- If the animal can't move, use the running-knot maneuver to restrain its head while you place a muzzle on it.
- If you're with another person, one of you can restrain the animal's head (by now already muzzled) and continue to soothe it, while the other administers first aid.

## Muzzling a dog

Before administering first aid to a conscious dog, it is vital that you muzzle it, especially if you're alone – even if you know the animal well and feel sure it won't bite. When a dog is in pain, it is always unpredictable and will probably bite.

- Use a commercial muzzle, such as a leather or nylon cage variety. Fit it over the animal's snout and fasten it behind the head. The "cage" allows the dog to breathe – and even vomit – easily.
- Don't use a muzzle made with compact material. The animal may panic or worse, be unable to breathe freely and even choke if it vomits. Always make sure that the animal can breathe freely after it has been muzzled.

---

1. Make sure you don't overtighten the knot in case you strangle the animal or cause a proptosis (when the eye pops out of its socket).

> Never muzzle an animal that has difficulty breathing
> or is unconscious.

Cats dislike being muzzled, and it may even be dangerous to try to muzzle an aggressive one. On the other hand, if a cat exhibits a great deal of aggressiveness, it may not be in any immediate danger. So try to lure it into a box instead, either by talking to it gently or using the bath towel technique (see page 26), then take it to the vet immediately.

---

### HOMEMADE MUZZLE

If commercial muzzles are unavailable, you can easily make one using whatever material comes to hand: a half-meter-long piece of gauze in your first-aid kit, for example, a strip of fabric, a pair of pantyhose, a necktie, or even a shoelace.

1. Make a loop in the center, large enough to slip over the dog's snout.
2. Stand behind the dog so that it can't bite you, and slip the loop over the snout.
3. Tighten the knot above the snout to prevent the material from slipping off. Make sure the knot is not too tight so that the dog can continue breathing freely.
4. Bring the loose ends together and crisscross under the animal's chin.
5. Pull the loose ends behind the ears and fasten them.

---

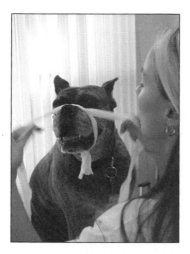
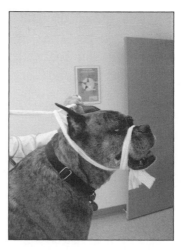

For short-snouted dogs, follow steps 1 to 5, then bring the loose ends from behind the head to the front, wrapping them around the snout one more time. Tie the loose ends either on top of the snout or behind the head.

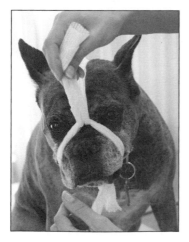
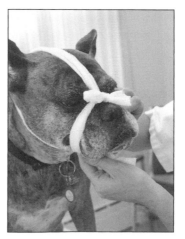

**Immobilizing an animal: the bath towel technique**
When an animal feels cornered, especially if it's already injured or otherwise vulnerable, its instinct is to become aggressive and fight back, compromising not only its own injuries, but also your personal safety. Therefore, use force sparingly if you want its cooperation. A bath towel or blanket – large enough to cover the entire animal – can be used to restrain the animal so that you can give it first aid or take it to the vet.
- Stay behind the animal and drape a bath towel or blanket over its body. Covering the animal will have a calming effect.
- Before picking up the animal (now covered with the towel) wrap your hand around its neck. Slowly wrap the towel around the body.
- Hold the animal in your arms and continue talking to it calmly. If you can manage, give it first aid; if not, then take the animal to the vet.
- If you're alone and the animal appears aggressive, disregard first aid (unless its injuries are life-threatening). The animal probably needs to be tranquilized. Instead, place it in a cardboard box or a cage and head for the vet.

**Immobilizing an animal using your own body**
This technique, which applies mostly to medium-size to large dogs, is used when an animal sustains minor, or non-life-threatening, injuries.
- Muzzle the dog before you immobilize it.
- Place your arm under and around the dog's neck, then grab and hold on firmly to the collar of your shirt. As a precaution, keep your face away from the dog's face.
- Curl your other arm around the dog's belly, pressing its body against your own.
- While you're immobilizing the dog, someone else can administer first aid. Keep talking to the animal reassuringly: this is also part of first aid.
- Try this technique only if you're perfectly comfortable with it, because it's not exactly risk-free. For example, if the animal you're trying to immobilize is a small breed, it can easily slip from your grasp and bite. If you hold its neck too tightly, you risk strangulation, even causing the eye to pop out of the sock-

et, a phenomenon called proptosis, common among flat-snouted dogs (Shih Tzu, bulldog, Yorkshire terrier).

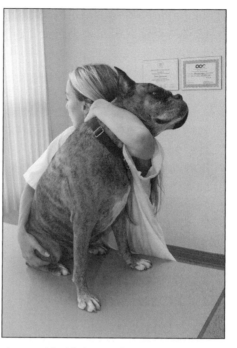

- For smaller dogs, you can use a muzzle or bath towel that you can wrap around its neck, like a shawl. This will prevent the dog from turning its head and biting you. If you're with another person, one of you can restrain the dog's head while the other administers first aid.

- If you can make the dog lie on its side willingly, place a bath towel over its neck in order to keep its head firmly on the ground, preventing it from biting. If there are two of you, one can sit behind the dog and hold down all its legs. Press the elbow closest to the animal's head on the bath towel to further restrain the head as the other person administers first aid.

> When immobilizing an animal, the key is to be gentle but firm.

## Getting an animal to lie on its side
- If it's a big dog, position yourself right beside it. Bend over the animal and put your arms under its body, grasping the front and hind legs closest to your own body.

- Gently lift the animal's legs so that its body can slide down your legs to the ground. Make sure the animal doesn't bang its head. Continue holding the legs while another person administers first aid.
- You can also apply this technique to a cat. Lay the animal gently on the ground, or a table, etc., but don't try to immobilize its neck with your forearm, because it can quickly turn around and bite you: cats are more flexible than dogs. Instead, grab the scruff of its neck with one hand – this won't hurt the cat – using the other to immobilize the hind legs.
- If the cat resists, or doesn't want to lie on its side because of injury, don't insist. Let it settle down as it pleases.
- Continue holding the cat by the scruff of its neck, and use the other hand to keep it down so another person can administer first aid.

Never lay an animal on its injured side.

If an animal resists efforts to immobilize it, leave it alone, or else it will bite you. In its already weakened state, the animal can panic easily, which will only worsen its condition.

## Transporting an injured animal

Taking an animal to the veterinary clinic is just as crucial as giving it first aid, because an incorrect move can worsen its injuries and cause complications. An injured or seriously ill animal tends to react irrationally and unpredictably because it's hurting: it may bite or run off if you try to control or manipulate it. First and foremost, always muzzle an injured dog as a precautionary measure. If you need to transport an injured animal, here are the dos and don'ts:

- Manipulate the animal as little as possible. Instead, encourage it to lie on its side. If it hesitates, it's probably sustained a chest or lung injury. Let it settle down as it pleases.
- Always proceed gently. Any abrupt manipulation may cause internal bleeding and damage the soft tissues around a fracture. If the animal is in shock, cover it up to calm it down and keep it warm.
- Don't apply any pressure to the animal's stomach and avoid lifting an injured animal by holding its abdomen, especially if it has difficulty breathing or you suspect internal injuries.
- Minimize the animal's movements by placing it on a flat surface – rigid cardboard box, wooden door, screen door – and securing it with a rope or duct tape. This is imperative if you think the animal has back injuries.
- Don't let a seriously wounded animal (struck by a car, for example) walk or climb into a motor vehicle by itself. This may set off – or worsen – internal bleeding, as well as cause the animal to go into shock.

**Transporting a small animal**
Small animals are easy to carry: in a box, for example, or wrapped in a blanket and held in your arms.

It's perfectly all right to carry a cat in your arms, by holding the scruff of its neck if necessary. Wrapping it in a bath towel is not just reassuring for the cat, but also prevents you from being scratched.

**Transporting a medium-size to large dog**
This requires an entirely different technique.
- Wrap your arm around the dog's neck from below.
- If you suspect an abdominal wound, place the other arm around the hind legs and hold the dog tightly against your body before lifting it.

- If you suspect a leg wound, wrap one arm around its neck and slip the other under its belly. Hold the dog tightly against your body before lifting it.

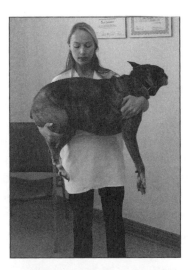

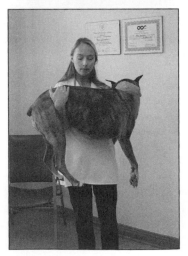

**Transporting a dog with two people**

Place the animal on a blanket and lift the latter by holding the corners. If the dog is very heavy, slide it on the blanket and drag it to the car. If the injured animal is unconscious, use the following technique:

- Position yourselves on the dog's uninjured side.
- Person A places one arm around the dog's neck and the other under its thorax, near the forelegs.
- Person B places one arm under the abdomen and the other under the pelvis, near the hind legs.

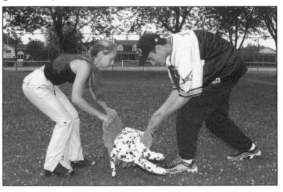

- Lift the animal at the same time.

## First Aid in Critical Situations

Certain emergencies require more complex knowledge and techniques: when an animal is unconscious or in a state of shock, for example, or when it experiences respiratory or cardiac arrest. In such cases, the ability to respond promptly – i.e., correctly assessing the animal's physical condition and applying appropriate resuscitation procedures – can make the difference between life and death.

### Loss of consciousness

Before undertaking CPR (cardiopulmonary resuscitation) or any similar life-saving maneuver, make sure that the animal is really unconscious. As a precaution, keep your face away from the animal and maintain a respectful distance. The animal may simply be sound asleep, especially if it's old, in which case it can leap up and bite if wakened by surprise. It's important, therefore, that you know how to assess an animal's state of consciousness. Try direct stimulation by using the following techniques.

### Assessing an animal's state of consciousness
- Speak softly to the animal.
- Clap your hands on each side of its head to see whether it reacts to noise: a conscious animal will move its ears or open its eyes, even if it's paralyzed.
- Try to waken the animal gently by stroking its flank, away from the head.
- Pinch the plantar pads so as to induce a reflex. The animal will automatically withdraw its leg if it feels the pinch. However, if it has a back injury, it may be unable to respond, even if conscious.
- If you get a response, the animal is breathing and its heart is functioning. Stay calm and let it wake up slowly. Check for injuries and give first aid as needed.
- If the animal fails to respond to any of the above stimuli, it is unconscious. Check to see if it's breathing, if the air passages are clear and the heart is beating. If not, start CPR to clear the air passages as well as restore breathing (artificial respiration) and circulation (external heart massage).

## Respiratory arrest
If the heart is beating but the animal is not breathing, you must clear the air passages and perform artificial respiration.

### Air passages
- Lay the animal on its side.
- Open its mouth and gently pull out its tongue, pushing it on one side. But be careful: even if the dog is unresponsive, it can bite as a reflex action.
- Align the head and neck. Handle the neck gently in case it is injured.
- Watch the chest movement and listen for breathing sounds. If you hear nothing and the air passages are clear, begin artificial respiration.

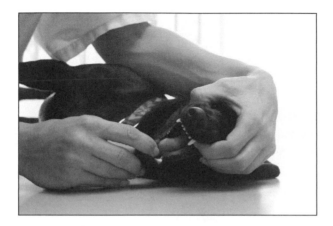

- Insert your fingers into the mouth and remove any saliva or vomit that might block the air passages. If you have to reach deeply into the animal's throat to recover a foreign object, make sure you don't confuse the obstruction with the "Adam's apple" so as not to damage or remove the latter by mistake.
- Pull the tongue to one side and stretch the neck to clear the air passages and stimulate breathing. An acupuncture point located in the middle of the upper lip (GV26) stimulates breathing. Activate it by pressing this spot with your nail.

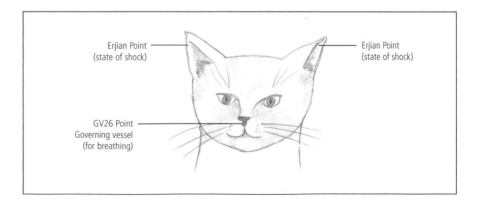

- If breathing doesn't resume after 10 seconds, begin artificial respiration.
- If the air passages are still blocked, try the Heimlich maneuver (see page 42).
- If breathing resumes, stop all maneuvers and allow the animal to rest quietly.
- Give necessary first aid.

### Artificial respiration

- Close the animal's muzzle with your hands, then place your mouth against its lips and blow three times, watching for the chest to rise. If it does, continue blowing 15 to 20 times per minute, or once every three seconds. Check regularly for a heartbeat, and to see if the animal has resumed breathing on its own.
- If you're dealing with a cat or a small flat-snouted dog, pinch the lips shut as you blow into the nostrils (20 to 25 times per minute, or once every two seconds). Check regularly for the heartbeat, and to see if the animal has resumed breathing on its own.
- Once the animal's lungs are filled with air, take a break and let them empty before blowing again. This will allow the air to be expelled, and encourage efficient return of blood to the heart.
- If the chest doesn't rise, it's because the air did not reach the lungs. Check the air passages again and remove any obstruction.

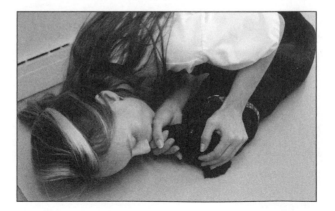

- If the heart is beating but the animal is not breathing on its own, continue artificial respiration (15 to 20 times per minute, or once every two to three seconds) for 20 minutes or until help arrives.
- Gently press the stomach to expel any air that might have entered because it hampers artificial respiration. But if you suspect internal bleeding, do not apply pressure to the abdomen.

## Cardiac arrest

Cardiac arrest interrupts the flow of blood and oxygen to the brain and other vital organs. When it occurs, you must act promptly – brain damage sets in within only three to four minutes – by massaging the heart in such a way as to help it resume pumping blood and oxygen. In addition, it's important to coordinate the chest compressions with artificial respiration; merely massaging the heart itself is a futile exercise.

The best way to assess cardiac function is checking for the heartbeat. You can do this by:

- Placing your ear on the left side of the animal's chest and listening for the heartbeat.
- Placing your hand on the inner thigh to feel the femoral pulse. If there's no pulse, then the heart has stopped. Keep in mind, however, that the pulse may be weak and hard to locate.

> Heart massage is useless if the air passages are blocked.
> Make sure they're clear before starting the dual task of
> chest compression and artificial respiration.

**External heart massage**

*Medium-size to large dogs*

- Place the dog on its right side (the heart is located on the left).
- Kneel down in front of the animal's chest.
- **Large dogs** (Bernese mountain dog, Great Dane, German shepherd, Labrador retriever, boxer, Dalmatian, etc.): Arrange the forelegs so that they are perpendicular to the body, as if the dog was standing. Flex its left elbow to a 90° angle to locate the position of the heart, just behind the elbow. Place both hands, one on top of the other, on the heart, then block the elbows. Compress the chest rhythmically: hold for a count of two, then release on a count of one. Repeat 80 to 100 times per minute. Apply enough pressure so as to lower the chest as much as 4 cm (1.5 in.) each time you compress.

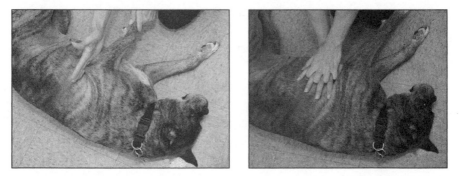

- **Medium-size dogs** (Shih Tzu, dachshund, terrier): Place your hands on each side of the thorax, just below the animal's elbow, at the spot where the chest is largest. Compress the chest with both hands, hold for a count of two, then release on a count of one, and so on, 120 times per minute. Apply enough pressure so as to lower the chest as much as 4 cm (1.5 in.) each time you compress (see page 37, upper photo).

### Cats, kittens and miniature dogs

- To locate the heart of a kitten, cat or miniature dog (Yorkshire terrier, miniature poodle), proceed in the same manner as above. Compress the chest with just one hand: fingers on one side and thumb on the other. Place the other hand on the animal's back for support. Compress the chest, hold for a count of two then release on a count of one, 120 times per minute. Lower the chest as much as 4 cm (1.5 in.) each time you compress.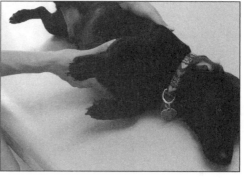
- If the pulse becomes perceptible or a strong heartbeat is felt, stop massaging and check for breathing.
- If the heartbeat resumes but the animal is still not breathing, stop massaging but continue artificial respiration until the animal breathes on its own.
- The routine is more effective if it's done by two first-aiders: while one compresses the chest, the other performs artificial respiration (one insufflation to every three to four chest compressions).
- If you're alone, blow twice for every 12 compressions. Check regularly for the pulse, heartbeat and breathing.
- If there are two first-aiders: one can continue CPR while the other drives to the veterinary hospital.

- It feels wonderful to have resuscitated an animal, but emergency care is far from over. Once the animal has resumed breathing, it must be seen by a vet without delay.

## State of shock

When the heart is unable to provide enough blood to the tissues, the cells are deprived of oxygen and die, sending the animal into a state of shock. Many factors contribute to this condition: trauma, severe burns (see page 81), severe pain, infection, blood loss, internal hemorrhage or bleeding (see page 111), fright or emotional stress (being pursued by another animal, a fight with another animal, incorrect treatment) and heart problems. A state of shock may be mild, medium or severe. Treatment varies depending on the gravity of the symptoms.

### Mild shock

The body can still compensate for the tissues' loss of blood and lack of oxygen.

| SYMPTOMS | FIRST AID |
|---|---|
| • Rapid heartbeat (see Normal Heart Rates, page 15). <br> • Excitement or unresponsiveness. <br> • Red and shiny gums. <br> • Hypothermia or fever if shock is caused by infection. <br> • Strong pulse (steady, distinct heartbeats are not hard to detect). <br> • Brief capillary refill time (one to two seconds) (see page 18). | • In the first stage of shock, you need only calm the animal down before the vital signs return to normal. <br> • If the animal experiences hypothermia (see page 121), keep it warm and take it to the vet. |

## Medium state of shock

The body has difficulty compensating for the inadequate supply of blood and oxygen.

| Symptoms | First aid |
|---|---|
| • Accelerated heartbeat (see Normal Heart Rates, page 15). <br> • Pale-colored gums. <br> • Capillary refill time longer than three seconds (see page 18). <br> • Weak pulse, hard to locate. <br> • Trembling. <br> • Hypothermia, cold limbs (see Normal Temperatures, page 12). <br> • Superficial and rapid breathing (but perhaps normal). <br> • Apathy and weakness. | • In some situations, you need only calm down and reassure the animal before its vital signs return to normal. <br> • Press the acupuncture point ("Erjian Point") located at the tip of the animal's ears (see illustration, page 33). <br> • If the animal has hypothermia (see page 121), give it first aid and consult a vet. <br> • Provide first aid for severe shock. |

### Severe state of shock

The body can no longer compensate for the lack of oxygen in organs and tissues. The animal is in critical danger.

| SYMPTOMS | FIRST AID |
|---|---|
| • Pale or bluish gums.<br>• Slow capillary refill time: more than three seconds (see page 18).<br>• Slow heartbeat (may be high or irregular and slowing down).<br>• Slow breathing (may be rapid, superficial or deep).<br>• Extremely weak pulse, difficult or impossible to detect.<br>• Hypothermia (see Normal Temperatures, page 12).<br>• Mental state deteriorating: going from apathy through stupor to coma (unconsciousness). | • If the animal is not breathing, try artificial respiration (see page 34).<br>• If there's no pulse or heartbeat, start CPR (see page 41).<br>• Control bleeding, if necessary (see page 107).<br>• Keep the animal warm; cover it with heated blankets and use hot-water bottles (see Normal Temperatures, page 12).<br>• Place the head lower than the body to maintain blood flow to the brain.<br>• ATTENTION: Do not lift the animal if you suspect neck or back injuries.<br>• Transport the animal to the vet immediately, taking all the required precautions into account. |

## CPR and State of Shock Flowchart

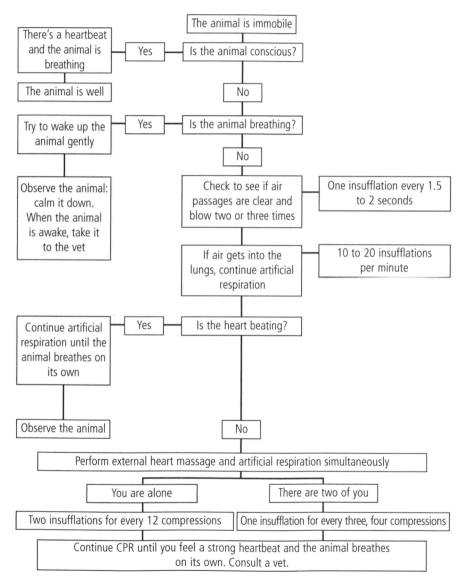

There's a heartbeat and the animal is breathing

The animal is immobile

— Yes — Is the animal conscious?

The animal is well

No

Try to wake up the animal gently — Yes — Is the animal breathing?

No

Observe the animal: calm it down. When the animal is awake, take it to the vet

Check to see if air passages are clear and blow two or three times — One insufflation every 1.5 to 2 seconds

If air gets into the lungs, continue artificial respiration — 10 to 20 insufflations per minute

Continue artificial respiration until the animal breathes on its own — Yes — Is the heart beating?

Observe the animal

No

Perform external heart massage and artificial respiration simultaneously

You are alone | There are two of you

Two insufflations for every 12 compressions | One insufflation for every three, four compressions

Continue CPR until you feel a strong heartbeat and the animal breathes on its own. Consult a vet.

## Choking

Choking caused by the presence of a foreign object in the trachea can lead to respiratory arrest within minutes, followed by cardiac arrest and death. If an animal starts to choke, perform the Heimlich maneuver on it immediately.

### Heimlich Maneuver

- **Large, heavy dogs:** If the dog is unconscious and heavy, it's impossible to perform the Heimlich maneuver while it's standing up. Lay the animal on the side, place your hand flat on its abdomen, behind the last rib, and compress it five times. If this doesn't work, lay the dog on its back and place your hand in the middle of the abdomen (plexus), then compress it five times with the heel of your hand pointing toward its head.

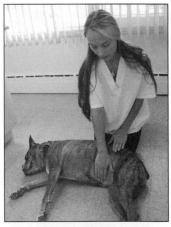

- **Medium-size dogs:** Hold the animal from behind, its head up and its back pressed against your legs. Place your hands on its abdomen, behind the last rib. Hold your hands together to make a fist. Do five abdominal thrusts upward (forming a "J"), gently but firmly.

    You can also perform the Heimlich maneuver by lifting the dog's pelvis, so that the head is pointed downward and the back is pressed against your legs, and by giving an abdominal thrust downward.

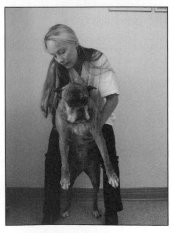

- **Small animals** (cat, kitten, miniature dogs): Follow the same steps as for medium-size dogs, but use the heel of your hand, rather than your fist, to do the abdominal thrusts.

If, after performing the Heimlich maneuver, the dog is still not breathing on its own, resume artificial respiration, blowing air twice into its lungs.

If the chest doesn't rise, then the air passages are still blocked. Repeat the Heimlich maneuver so as to dislodge the foreign object, followed by artificial respiration, up to 10 to 15 times per minute (see page 34), until the animal resumes breathing on its own.

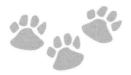

## Chapter 3
## BIRTHING COMPLICATIONS
## AND FIRST AID
## FOR NEWBORN ANIMALS

Generally speaking, cats and dogs don't need our help when giving birth. You need only provide a quiet, clean area, softly lit, away from distractions, and comfortable bedding (blankets and newspapers). Delivery often occurs when you least expect it, even during your absence.

Some animals, however, will need comforting, especially if it's their first time. The mother-to-be tends to be nervous and confused about what to do. Keeping the animal company helps to calm her down. But it's important that only one person stay with the animal, because a constant coming-and-going will only increase its anxiety and may even delay the birth.

Just before it goes into labor, a dog tends to turn round and round looking for a nest. Its appetite decreases and, 24 hours before giving birth, its body temperature drops to 37.7°C (100°F).

A cat, on the other hand, meows constantly to attract attention, looking for comfort and guidance. The animal tends to take refuge inside a closet, under a bed or table, for a place to give birth.

Acquaint the expectant mother with the delivery area several weeks before the due date. Choose a room familiar to the animal, where it feels secure, and give it a box filled with blankets so that it can settle down comfortably. This way, the animal will feel perfectly at home when the time comes.

## Three Phases of the Birthing Process

The three phases of birthing are dilation of the cervix, the delivery itself and the first few minutes of life. Familiarize yourself with the characteristics of each, so that you can detect potential complications as early as possible.

Many factors can cause complications during the birth cycle. The most common are: absence of contractions (stillborn); weak contractions; a distracting environment; noise, commotion during delivery; the presence of other animals; abnormal birth canal; excessively large fetus; twins (two fetuses in the same amniotic cavity); wrong fetal position (limbs first, rather than head); delayed delivery (gestation lasting more than 62 to 64 days); uterine torsion.

### Phase One
Phase One normally lasts 6 to 12 hours and is characterized by uterine contractions that are invisible because of the dilated cervix. The only sign of imminent delivery is the mother's unusual behavior: the animal is restless, unable to find a comfortable position, and tends to pant, constantly pacing back and forth.

### Potential complications
If, after 12 hours, the female is still in Phase One, consult a vet.

## Phase Two

It lasts three to six hours (10 to 12 hours if the animal is disturbed). In addition to panting, Phase Two is characterized by visible, faster and stronger abdominal contractions.

Delivery should take place less than an hour into Phase Two. The first kitten or puppy normally appears either head or tail end first. If contractions are strong, the rest of the litter should follow, one by one, at 10- to 30-minute intervals. If contractions are weak, up to four to six hours will elapse between births. No contractions occur during the pauses, which is normal.

## Potential complications

Many complications can arise at the birthing stage. So be vigilant!

## Symptoms

- Contractions in quick succession, but no fetus appears.
- Contractions lasting more than 30 minutes before delivery occurs.
- Lethargy, weakness and pale-colored gums (state of shock).
- Bleeding prior to delivery.
- Gestation lasting more than 62-64 days.
- Dark-colored and malodorous vaginal discharge.

## First aid

- Should the fetus remain stuck in the birth canal for five to 10 minutes, rub the animal's abdomen to stimulate contractions.
- If the fetus is part way out, you can help the mother expel it completely by pulling gently on the fetus during contractions, using a lubricant gel and a clean cloth or gauze sponge.
- If only the head is out, do not pull, but stimulate contractions by rubbing the abdomen. If you pull on the fetus in the absence of a contraction, you'll risk decapitating the fetus and injuring the mother.

## Phase Three

Immediately or within minutes of birth the placenta is expelled, and the mother normally ingurgitates it, entirely or in part. Nutrient-rich, the placenta will help with the postpartum recovery.

The female usually takes care of her newborn following birthing. After sectioning the umbilical cord with her teeth, she licks her young vigorously to stimulate breathing and its sucking instinct. Kittens and puppies are highly sensitive to temperature change, requiring heat as intense as 32.2°C (90°F) during the first week of life. This is why the mother keeps her offspring close to her body. As well, the babies need to receive the colostrum, the first milk secretion after birth, rich in maternal antibodies.

### Potential complications

If the female is too exhausted to look after her newborn, allow her to rest, and give the kitten or puppy the necessary care yourself.

### First aid for the newborn animal

- Remove the placenta membranes covering the newborn's body, face and mouth.
- Gently wipe mucus from the mouth and nose.
- Hold the puppy or kitten with its head pointed downward to drive any fluid out of its lungs.
- If the mother fails to lick and clean its offspring to stimulate breathing, cover the newborn in a towel or soft cloth and rub it gently for a few minutes. This will keep it warm and stimulate breathing.
- If the kitten doesn't start breathing quickly after being rubbed, give it artificial respiration. Blow gently, because very little air is needed to fill its tiny lungs.
- Don't give up after only a few attempts at stimulation and artificial respiration. Resuscitation maneuvers often last five to 10 minutes before a newborn will respond.

- Once it has started breathing, return the newborn to its mother so it can nurse and keep warm.
- If the newborn is breathing and its skin is pink, you may proceed to cut the umbilical cord. Tie two strips of dental floss around the cord: the first about 2.5 cm (1 in.) from the animal's body, and the second strip about 2.5 cm from the first. Cut the umbilical cord between the two strips, using scissors that have been disinfected with alcohol. Gently apply iodine on the animal's end of the umbilical cord. Do not pull on it, or you'll risk causing an umbilical hernia.

## Common Complications at the End of Pregnancy and After Birth

The female cat and dog may suffer from various complications during or following pregnancy. Learn about them so you can intervene in time and avoid serious problems.

### Eclampsia

Eclampsia occurs in the final weeks of pregnancy or during the lactation period, two or three weeks following birth, when the mother has difficulty maintaining a good calcium balance in the blood. It stems from calcium deficiency and is characterized by involuntary muscular spasms (in the limbs or a group of muscles), convulsions and fever.

### First aid

- Eclampsia requires prompt intervention. You must take the animal to a vet immediately.
- If this complication occurs at the time of birth, provide the puppies or kittens with a substitute for their mother's milk.

- You can prevent eclampsia by feeding the mother puppy or kitten food – easily available at a vet's office – during pregnancy and throughout the lactation period.
- If you prepare the food yourself, make sure to include green vegetables and calcium, as well as a vitamin supplement.

## Mastitis

Mastitis is an inflammation of the mammary glands, perhaps a result of wounds inflicted by kittens and puppies during nursing, or an unclean environment.

## Symptoms

- Mammary glands and nipples swollen and sensitive to the touch.
- Blood and pus discharge.
- Fever.
- Mother's refusal to nurse its offspring.

## First aid

- Clean the mammary glands with warm water and an antiseptic soap. Rinse thoroughly.
- Apply hot compresses: warm up a hot-or-cold gel pack – or a bag of uncooked rice – in the microwave oven for a minute or two and wrap in a towel to avoid burning. This measure will help to decongest the mammary glands and reduce their sensitivity.
- See a vet.

## Uterine prolapse

Uterine prolapse is a condition that causes a female's uterus to slide into the vagina shortly after it has given birth. You will notice a red mass, either large or small, appearing from the vulva; the affected tissues are swollen, may even dry up and die.

## First aid

- Clean the exposed tissues delicately with warm water.
- Dab a sterile gauze pad with a lubricant gel and place it on the tissues, pushing them back into the vagina, gently but firmly.
- If the prolapse is too large or you cannot replace the tissues in their normal position, keep them moist with lubricant gel and water, wrapping them in sterile gauze.
- Prevent the animal from mutilating itself. Put an Elizabethan collar (a plastic, cone-shaped device) around its neck.
- This is an emergency: the affected animal is susceptible to toxic septicemia and uterine necrosis. Consult a vet as soon as possible.

## After an Animal is Born

Once the female has given birth, it requires much less attention. But it's important that you provide an environment conducive to proper care. The following steps are a good start:

- Place the new family in a quiet area. A noisy environment will prompt them to move elsewhere.
- Leave food and water within reach so the mother can feed herself and be with her young. A female is often reluctant to leave her offspring behind, some even abstain from eating.
- Give the mother nutrient-rich puppy or kitten food (easily available at a vet's office) throughout the lactation period.
- Provide the new family with a comfortable and warm nest, complete with blankets, towels or newspapers to conserve heat.
- The female will have brownish-red or green vaginal discharge one to four weeks following birth. These secretions are perfectly normal. But if they turn red or yellow (pus) and are malodorous, consult a vet.

## Normal behavior

Being familiar with a newborn's normal behavior helps you detect potential problems. Kittens and puppies have very similar characteristics and needs at birth:

- They can crawl and stand at birth.
- Kittens and puppies typically start to shiver a week after birth, a sign that their bodies are starting to respond and adapt to temperature changes. But they still require their mother's warmth to maintain a stable, adequate body temperature throughout the first month of life – between 34.4 and 37.2°C (94 – 99°F) for weeks 1 and 2, and between 36 and 37.7°C (97 – 100°F) for weeks 3 and 4. Once the critical first month has passed, kittens and puppies can maintain adequate body temperature, between 37.7 and 38°C (100 – 101°F), by themselves.
- They need their mother's assistance in stimulating urination and defecation. The female instinctively ingurgitates its offspring's excreta, thus eliminating odors and keeping potential predators away.
- The umbilical cord will dry up and fall off between two and three days after birth.
- A newborn breathes 15 to 35 times per minute.
- The auditory canals open between the sixth and 14th day for kittens, and between the 13th and 17th for puppies.
- Kittens open their eyes between the 10th and 14th day (blue eyes) and their vision becomes clear between the 22nd and 28th day. Puppies open their eyes between the first and third week.
- Kittens generally double their weight in the first week. Weight increase is harder to predict for puppies, because it depends on the breed.
- Kittens walk at 21 days; puppies at 21 to 28 days.

## Orphaned puppies or kittens

Occasionally, a female will die during birth or shortly thereafter, leaving tiny and vulnerable orphans behind. Too often this means that the kittens or puppies will not survive. But the truth is, there's nothing inevitable about it, because humans are perfectly capable of looking after them properly.

An orphan puppy or kitten mainly requires warmth and food. Make sure you provide them, first and foremost, with a warm environment and an adequate substitute for mother's milk.

| AMBIENT TEMPERATURES FOR KITTENS AND PUPPIES | | |
|---|---|---|
| AGE | AMBIENT TEMPERATURES | |
| **Kitten** | | |
| Up to 7 days | 80 to 92°F | 26.6 to 33.3°C |
| 8 to 14 days | 80 to 85°F | 26.6 to 29.4°C |
| 15 – 28 days | 80°F | 26.6°C |
| 29 – 35 days | 75°F | 23.8°C |
| Over 35 days | 70°F | 21.1°C |
| **Puppy** | | |
| Up to 5 days | 85 to 90°F | 29.4 to 32.2°C |
| 6 to 20 days | 80°F | 26.6°C |
| 21 – 28 days | 78°F | 25.5°C |
| 29 – 35 days | 75°F | 23.8°C |
| Over 35 days | 70°F | 21.1°C |

Wrap the orphan in blankets and place it in a cardboard or wooden box (never metal) insulated with paper at the bottom. Heat is crucial during the first week of life. Keep the animal warm with hot-water bottles, or a gel pack, pre-heated for a minute or two in the microwave oven, then wrapped in a towel.

Do not place a newborn animal on a direct heat source because it may get badly burned. Always add a layer of insulation – a towel or blanket – between the heat source and the kittens or puppies.

Heating pads are very useful, because you can control the heat and maintain a comfortable ambient temperature. Again, never place the orphan directly on a heating pad, always cover it with thick towels or a blanket first.

## Food for newborns

Feeding a newborn puppy or kitten requires special care. The diet must be healthy, rich in nutrients, and dispensed several times a day, on a strict schedule. It's crucial that you use top-quality ingredients when preparing the mother's milk substitute and scrupulously observe basic hygiene rules. The slightest carelessness may lead to serious health problems, such as diarrhea, and even death.

Keep the formula in the refrigerator (up to two days) and heat only the portion needed for each feed. Use a pet-nurser bottle, usually included in a first-aid kit or available at a vet's office. Avoid using an eyedropper, because the puppy or kitten cannot suck at it and the milk might accidentally get drawn into the lungs.

The prescribed daily milk portion corresponds to 25 percent of the animal's weight. Feed it six times a day during the first two weeks, then four times a day afterward, until it is weaned.

## MOTHER'S MILK SUBSTITUTE FOR KITTENS AND PUPPIES

| | |
|---|---|
| 240 ml (8 oz) | Homogenized or evaporated milk (if you use evaporated milk, dilute two parts milk in one part water). Mother's milk substitutes are also available at a vet's office. |
| 5 ml (1 teaspoon) | Canola oil |
| 1 drop | Multivitamins for humans (or for kittens) |
| 2 | Egg yolks |
| 5 ml (1 teaspoon) | Corn syrup |

Put all ingredients in a mixer and warm the milk before each feeding.

### After each feed
Help the tiny animal to burp after each feed. Then wash its abdomen and genitals with warm water to stimulate urination and defecation. Gently dry then rub the animal.

### Weaning kittens and puppies
You can start weaning a kitten or a puppy as early as the fourth week. Here's how:

- Add 5 to 10 ml (1 to 2 teaspoons) of Pablum, a rice cereal for human consumption, to each meal's portion of the formula.
- At five weeks, encourage the animal to lick the Pablum-added formula from a dish. Add enough Pablum to get a thick consistency.
- At six weeks, start giving kitten or puppy food, dipped in or mixed with water and Pablum-added formula. Encourage the animal to eat from a dish.
- From six to eight weeks, gradually reduce the amount of formula and Pablum until they are eating only the kitten or puppy food.

## Hypoglycemia in kittens and puppies

Kittens and puppies are especially prone to developing hypoglycemia. This is because they are young and growing and therefore need lots of food, which is in turn rapidly metabolized.

| CAUSES | SYMPTOMS |
|---|---|
| • Mother doesn't produce sufficient milk.<br>• Newborn receives an insufficient amount of food (not more than twice a day).<br>• Presence of intestinal worms. | • Weakness.<br>• Wobbly gait.<br>• Disorientation.<br>• Shivering.<br>• Epilepsy.<br>• Unconsciousness. |

Hypoglycemia in kittens and puppies is treated in the same manner as for adult animals (see Hypoglycemia, page 120). To prevent it, feed the kittens and puppies four to six times a day with especially prepared, top-quality food.

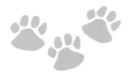

# Chapter 4
# POISONING

**N**aturally curious and always hungry, every animal, especially dogs, is interested in whatever's within reach. This helps explain the high number of pet poisonings. In most cases, improperly stored domestic products are the culprits. That's why it's important to keep all potentially harmful products (cleaning or other) away from your pet.

## Common Toxic Products and Basic First Aid

There is a long list of toxic substances as far as your pet is concerned; however, the following products are those an animal is most likely to encounter. Generally, poisoning provokes one or more of the symptoms noted below. While basic first aid for a poisoned animal is usually the same no matter what the poison source, certain products cause specific symptoms or require special treatment. These will be discussed in separate sections.

| CAUSES | SYMPTOMS |
|---|---|
| • Alcohol.<br>• Antifreeze (windshield wiper fluid).<br>• Broken glass.<br>• Chocolate.<br>• Cosmetics.<br>• Gasoline, oil, petroleum products.<br>• Household cleaning agents.<br>• Household garbage.<br>• Household plants.<br>• Insecticides, herbicides.<br>• Medication and drugs (prescription drugs, narcotics, illegal drugs).<br>• Paint.<br>• Plastic.<br>• Tylenol (acetaminophen) or aspirin.<br>• Wild plants (poisonous mushrooms, for example). | One or more of the following symptoms may be observed. Some can lead to death.<br>• Abdominal pain.<br>• Convulsions.<br>• Depression.<br>• Diarrhea.<br>• Excessive salivation.<br>• Excitability.<br>• Lack of coordination.<br>• Shock.<br>• Vomiting.<br>• Weakness. |

**First aid**
- Locate the source of poisoning and read the label for the recommended antidote.
- Look for clues to identify the product your pet may have swallowed: torn or open garbage bags or container, antifreeze or oil, chocolate wrappings, etc.
- If the animal is conscious and able to swallow, and if the toxic substance was ingested no longer than three hours previously, induce vomiting.
- Once the animal has vomited, give it activated carbon (included in your first-aid kit or available at the pharmacy): 1 to 4 g per kilogram/2.2 pounds of pet's weight, with water.
- Call a veterinarian.

## Inducing Vomiting

Inducing vomiting allows the stomach to expel toxic substances before they can be absorbed by the body. Give the poisoned pet one or other of the following:

- Salt (5 ml/ 1 teaspoon) at the back of the mouth, on the tongue.
- Hydrogen peroxide (3%) by mouth, according to the animal's weight: a 15-ml dose (1 tablespoon) per 6.8 to 9 kilograms (15 to 20 pounds.). Repeat once, if necessary.

### When not to induce vomiting

Do not induce vomiting if:

- The animal is lethargic, weak or depressed. Take it to the vet immediately.
- The animal is unconscious. Check its vital signs and perform cardiopulmonary resuscitation (CPR) if necessary.
- The animal suffers from epilepsy.
- The label on the toxic product advises against induced vomiting.
- The poison source is an acid or alkaline substance, a petroleum derivative or cleaning agent. Vomiting would further expose the esophagus to the toxic substance and cause additional tissue damage.
- The substance was ingested more than three hours previously.

## Toxic Household Products

A number of domestic products contain highly toxic chemicals that can burn, harm the nervous system, and even lead to death if appropriate first aid is not quickly administered.

If a herbicide or insecticide comes in contact with an animal's skin, rinse the lesion with water, then clean it with dishwashing soap. Shave the affected area if the product has penetrated the fur. If the animal has swallowed the material, read the product label for first-aid instructions. This is essential because herbicides and insecticides may contain ingredients such as acid, nitrates, phenol, hormones, phosphates, chloro-hydrocarbon, which require different treatment. If you can't identify the product, give the animal activated carbon and contact your local poison center and the veterinarian.

### Boric acid

Boric acid irritates the skin on contact; if ingested, it can damage the kidneys and liver. Cats or dogs – especially kittens and puppies – that play with ant traps can break them open and swallow the contents. If you find a broken or chewed up container, or see your pet playing with an ant trap, it has probably eaten boric acid.

| CAUSE | SYMPTOMS |
|---|---|
| • Ingestion of boric acid (ant traps, denture-cleaning products). | • Diarrhea.<br>• Muscular weakness.<br>• Ataxia (unsteadiness).<br>• Convulsions.<br>• Trembling.<br>• Depression.<br>• Blood in the urine.<br>• Swelling of the lips and skin.<br>• Skin irritation (after having chewed on the container). |

**First aid**

- Baking soda mixed with water (half and half) to neutralize the poison.
- Activated carbon (1 to 4 g per kilogram/2.2 pounds of pet weight).
- Contact your vet immediately.
- Bring the container with you.

## Ethylene glycol (Antifreeze)

Ethylene glycol is used as an antifreeze in winter and a coolant in summer for automobile engines. It can also be found in industrial solvents, rust removal products, liquids used to develop color photos and heat-activating liquids. As little as 2 to 4 ml per kilogram ($^1/_2$ to 1 teaspoon per 2.2 pounds) for cats and 5 ml per kilogram (1 teaspoon per 2.2 pounds) for dogs can cause kidney failure or death.

| CAUSES | SYMPTOMS |
|---|---|
| <ul><li>Pet attracted by ethylene glycol's sweet taste.</li><li>Cat sheltering under the hood of a car to keep warm near the engine licks antifreeze spills.</li><li>Animal has torn open a chemical product.</li></ul> | Up to four hours following ingestion:<ul><li>Lack of coordination.</li><li>Rapid heartbeat and breathing.</li><li>Drinking large quantities of water.</li><li>Dehydration.</li></ul>From four to six hours following ingestion:<ul><li>Loss of appetite.</li><li>Depression.</li><li>Vomiting.</li><li>Hypothermia.</li><li>Rapid breathing.</li><li>Kidney failure.</li><li>Coma.</li></ul> |

**First aid**
- If the ingestion took place no longer than four hours earlier, give the animal activated carbon according to its weight: 1 to 4 g per kilogram/2.2 pounds, with water.
- Act promptly: Your pet's life is in danger!
- See your vet immediately.

## Naphthalene

Naphthalene (petroleum hydrocarbon), commonly used in mothballs, is a volatile substance that is toxic both to humans and animals. Poisoning can occur by inhalation or through skin contact.

Many people use naphthalene in closets, wardrobes and drawers to eliminate moths and other insects.

Cats are more likely to be poisoned by naphthalene because they like to hide and sleep in enclosed spaces where the product is often used. The poisoned animal can develop hemolytic anemia (destruction of red blood cells) and methemoglobinemia (in which blood oxygen is dangerously reduced), especially in the kidneys and liver, leading to death. Therefore, it's a good idea to dispose of all naphthalene-based products found in the home.

| CAUSE | SYMPTOMS |
|---|---|
| • Contact with naphthalene. | • Pet smells of naphthalene.<br>• Bad breath.<br>• Pale gums.<br>• Weakness.<br>• Loss of appetite. |

**First aid**
- Administer activated carbon (1 to 4 g per kilogram/2.2 pounds).
- See a vet immediately. Your pet's life is in danger.

## Acids, alkaline substances or petroleum derivatives

Cleaning agents, beauty products, insecticides and herbicides contain toxic substances that fall into three main categories: acids, alkaline substances and petroleum derivatives. Appropriate first aid given will depend on the ingested product. That is why it's important to correctly identify the product that has poisoned your pet.

| CAUSES | SYMPTOMS |
|---|---|
| • Ingestion of acid (read the label): household cleaning agents, beauty products, nail polish remover, boric acid (ant traps), acetone, insecticides, herbicides, etc. <br> • Ingestion of an alkali (read the label): caustic cleaners (for example, drain decloggers), household cleaning agents, soaps, paint, herbicides, etc. <br> • Ingestion of a petroleum derivative: motor oil, varnish, rubber, turpentine, disinfectants, rubbing alcohol, etc. | • Pet can show one or more of the previously cited symptoms. |

## First aid

If you don't know what type of product (acid, alkali or petroleum derivative) was ingested, contact a poison-control center or a veterinarian. You'll be asked for the following information: the name of the product (have the container with its active ingredients list handy); the approximate time the poison was ingested; and the animal's symptoms.

In poisoning cases, the faster treatment is given – either by inducing vomiting or administering products that will dilute or neutralize the toxic substance – the better the animal's chances of survival. Although such measures can reduce the poison's toxic effects, a trip to the vet is essential.

If you know the type of substance ingested, administer the recommended first aid immediately, then contact your vet.

- **Acid:** Administer 5 to 10 ml (1 to 2 teaspoons) of baking soda, diluted in 125 ml (½ cup) of water, to help neutralize the poison. Next, give the animal activated carbon (1 to 4 g per kilogram/2.2 pounds).
- **Alkali:** Administer an acid product, such as lemon juice or vinegar with water (half and half) to help neutralize the poison. Follow up with activated carbon (1 to 4 g per kilogram of the pet's weight).
- **Petroleum derivative:** Have the animal drink milk or water to dilute the poison. Within four hours after the poisoning occurs, give the pet activated carbon (1 to 4 g per kilogram/2.2 pounds) or mineral oil (15 to 30 ml/ 1 to 2 tablespoons for a dog and 5 to 10 ml/ 1 to 2 teaspoons for a cat) diluted in milk or water. The oil slows down the body's absorption of the toxic substance.

## Medications, Narcotics and Stimulants

Pets are regularly poisoned by medications, narcotics and stimulants. In most cases, such incidents are the result of negligence or ignorance and could easily have been avoided.

But they should always be taken seriously because the consequences are serious, even putting an animal's life at risk. This is why it's important that such products be kept out of reach.

### Acetaminophen

Most cases of acetaminophen poisoning (in Tylenol, for example) occur because a well-intentioned pet owner has administered the medication to a pet or because a dog has chewed on the tablet container.

Cats are more susceptible to acetaminophen poisoning than dogs because their livers cannot metabolize the medication. The product destroys red blood cells. A normal dose of 325 mg of acetaminophen is toxic for a cat and a further 325-mg dose 24 hours later can be fatal.

| CAUSE | SYMPTOMS |
|---|---|
| • Ingestion of acetaminophen. | • Anemia: check the gums. Are they pale pink or white? <br> • Breathing difficulty occurring four to 12 hours after ingestion. <br> • Swelling of the face and paws. <br> • Itching. <br> • Lack of appetite. <br> • Depression. <br> • Jaundice: occurs from two to seven days after ingestion. |

**First aid**
- If ingestion took place less than four hours earlier, induce vomiting (see page 59).
- Give the animal activated carbon relative to its weight (1 to 4 g per kilogram/2.2 pounds) and water.
- Contact your vet immediately so the animal can be given an antidote and appropriate care.

In cases of poisoning by illegal drugs, the pet owner may hesitate to contact a veterinarian. However, since the animal's medical file is confidential, there is no reason not to seek professional care. Your pet's life may depend on it.

## Amphetamines

Amphetamines are found in appetite suppressants and decongestants. Amphetamine poisoning affects the nervous system.

| CAUSE | SYMPTOMS |
|---|---|
| • Ingestion of appetite suppressant, decongestants or any other substance containing amphetamines. | • Agitation.<br>• Change in behavior, hyperactivity.<br>• Kidney failure.<br>• Fever.<br>• Rapid breathing (See Normal Respiratory Rates, page 13).<br>• Accelerated heartbeat (See Normal Heart Rates, page 15).<br>• Trembling, convulsions.<br>• Shock.<br>• Dilation of the pupils. |

### First aid

*If the animal has ingested a large number of pills less than two hours earlier and shows no symptom of intoxication:*
• Induce vomiting (see page 59).
• Take the animal to the vet immediately.

*If the animal shows signs of intoxication:*
• Do not induce vomiting.
• Be ready to perform cardiopulmonary resuscitation.
• Take the animal to the vet immediately.

## Chocolate

Chocolate contains theobromine and caffeine. Both stimulate the nervous system and are toxic for animals. Theobromine brings on excessive secretion of epinephrine (adrenaline) which increases an animal's heart rate and can trigger an arrhythmia. A dose of only 100 to 200 mg/kg of caffeine or theobromine is fatal. A small dog weighing one to two kilograms (2.2 to 4.4 pounds) can die after eating only 30 g (one ounce) of dark chocolate. It is not uncommon for dogs to eat stimulating medicines accidentally, but the ingestion of chocolate is even more frequent, especially during the holiday season.

---

### COMMON SOURCES OF THEOBROMINE

Chocolate contains between 80 and 85 percent theobromine and 15 to 20 percent caffeine. Theobromine levels in coffee and chocolate in various forms:

Regular coffee (6-10 mg per 30 g)
Cooking chocolate, unsweetened (400 mg per 30 g)
Milk chocolate (50 mg per 30 g)
Dark chocolate (150 mg per 30 g)
Cocoa beans (contain 4-8 g per 30 g)
Caffeine tablets (100-200 mg/pill)
Tea (contains caffeine)

---

| CAUSE | SYMPTOMS |
|---|---|
| • Ingestion of chocolate, coffee or tea. | • Agitation, hyperactivity (less than two hours after ingestion).<br>• Excessive urination.<br>• Vomiting.<br>• Diarrhea.<br>• Stiffness, trembling and convulsions.<br>• Breathing difficulty and increased heart rate (see Normal Heart Rates, page 15).<br>• Fever (see Hyperthermia, page 118).<br>• Coma. |

**First aid**
- If the pet has ingested chocolate or coffee within the last four hours and shows no symptom of poisoning other than diarrhea, induce vomiting (see page 59) and administer a dose of activated carbon geared to its weight (1 to 4 g per kilogram or 2.2 pounds). Dilute in water.
- If the animal shows signs of poisoning, do not induce vomiting. If it's able to swallow, administer activated carbon based on its weight (1 to 4 g per kilogram/2.2 pounds). Dilute in water.
- Contact a vet immediately. Medication to stabilize the heart and prevent shock will be required.

> Keep all foods containing chocolate out of the reach of pets. Children should be taught not to give chocolate or sweets to pets.

## Cocaine

Cocaine is a powerful drug that is quickly absorbed by the body after inhalation or ingestion. Therefore, if your pet has ingested cocaine, you must act promptly because its life could be in danger.

| CAUSE | SYMPTOMS |
|---|---|
| • Cocaine ingestion. | • Agitation.<br>• Trembling.<br>• Fever.<br>• Respiratory arrest.<br>• Cardiac arrest. |

### First aid

*If the animal is conscious:*
- Induce vomiting (see page 59).
- Administer activated carbon.
- Be ready to perform cardiopulmonary resuscitation (CPR).
- Take it to the vet immediately.

*If the animal is unconscious:*
- Check vital signs and begin CPR, if necessary.
- Take the pet to the vet immediately.

## Marijuana and hashish

Marijuana and hashish are drugs derived from the leaves, stems and flowers of Indian hemp or cannabis. Poisoning can result from inhaling the smoke or ingesting a joint (marijuana cigarette), or even from baked foods that have been spiked with the drug. In general, cats are poisoned by inhaling smoke from a marijuana cigarette. Dogs, typically hungry, are more likely to ingest the drug.

| CAUSE | SYMPTOMS |
|---|---|
| • Marijuana absorption. | • Change in behavior, hyperactivity.<br>• Lack of coordination, muscular weakness.<br>• Stupor, extreme apathy.<br>• Dilated pupils.<br>• Vomiting.<br>• Depression.<br>• Hypothermia or hyperthermia.<br>• Panting.<br>• Slow heartbeat.<br>• Trembling and convulsions. |

**First aid**

Do not induce vomiting if the animal is lethargic and depressed or if it has already vomited. This can cause choking. Take it to a vet immediately. Check vital signs and be ready to perform cardiopulmonary resuscitation (CPR).

*If the poisoning occurred less than an hour earlier:*
- Induce vomiting (see page 59).
- After the animal has vomited, give it activated carbon in accordance with its weight: 1 to 4 g per kilogram/ 2.2 pounds, with water. Activated carbon absorbs toxins in the digestive system, slowing their absorption by the body.
- Contact a vet.

*If the poisoning occurred more than an hour earlier:*
- Do not induce vomiting.
- Administer activated carbon.
- Contact a vet.

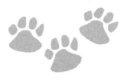

# Chapter 5
# EMERGENCY BASICS

## Allergic Reactions

A pet may develop allergies to many household products, but allergic reactions are generally caused by vaccinations or insect bites and stings (from bee, wasp, yellow jacket, hornet, red ants, spiders). Reactions range from minor – with localized swelling – to severe, even causing death from anaphylactic shock.

An allergic reaction to a vaccination may manifest itself by a light swelling around the injection site, but it can be much more severe, with similar symptoms as those caused by insect and spider bites or stings. The same first-aid techniques apply in both cases.

When you take your pet for its shots, do so early in the day. The vet's office will still be open if the animal later develops allergic symptoms.

## Minor allergic reaction
It is localized and generally disappears within a few hours.

| CAUSES | SYMPTOM |
|---|---|
| • Insect bites and stings.<br>• Vaccination. | • Swelling (small bump) painful to the touch, usually around hairless areas (snout, paws, face). |

**First aid**
- Remove the sting with a credit card or fingernail. Don't pinch, you'll risk embedding it further. A sting will continue to emit poison for up to three minutes while it remains in the animal's skin.
- Clean the affected area with disinfectant soap.
- Relieve the burning sensation by applying baking soda to the affected area for bee stings, and vinegar for wasp stings.
- Apply ice cubes to diminish pain.

## Medium allergic reaction

A medium allergic reaction is obviously more serious, with symptoms (as noted above) spreading over the entire affected region. The same first-aid procedure applies.

| CAUSES | SYMPTOMS |
|---|---|
| • Insect bites and stings.<br>• Vaccination. | • Entire leg affected or swollen face.<br>• Painful to the touch.<br>• Redness.<br>• Skin eruption and bumps around sting (may spread to other areas). |

**First aid**

- Same first-aid procedure as for light allergic reaction.
- If the animal has difficulty breathing and you can't get to a vet, give it an anti-histamine (Benadryl, for example), if possible, in syrup rather than tablet form. Syrup is easier to swallow and is absorbed as soon as it touches the tongue and the gums. If the pet resists the medication, administer a small dose at a time, making sure it comes in contact with both tongue and gums.
- Take the animal to a vet as soon as possible. If your pet is due for vaccinations, it is wise to observe and stay with your pet for a few hours in case there is an allergic reaction.

---

**DIPHENHYDRAMINE HYDROCHLORIDE (BENADRYL) DOSAGE**

Small dogs or cats, under 13.5 kilograms (30 pounds): 10 mg
Dogs 13.5 – 22.5 kilograms (30-50 pounds): 25 mg
Dogs over 22.5 kilograms (over 50 pounds): 50 mg

---

## Severe allergic reaction: anaphylactic shock

A severe systemic reaction (called anaphylactic shock) can occur within 15 minutes after the body has been infected with the venom of a spider, snake or insect. Death may occur in less than an hour. On rare occasions, vaccinations will produce the same effect.

| CAUSES | SYMPTOMS |
|---|---|
| • Insect bites and stings.<br>• Vaccination. | **Dogs**<br>• Breathing difficulty.<br>• Convulsions.<br>• Defecation, urination.<br>• Muscle weakness.<br>• Swelling (neck, face or legs).<br>• Vomiting.<br><br>**Cats**<br>• Breathing difficulty.<br>• Collapse.<br>• Itching.<br>• Lack of coordination.<br>• Salivation.<br>• Swelling on neck. |

**First aid**

- Check vital signs and perform CPR, if necessary (see page 41).
- If the animal is conscious, is not vomiting, and can swallow: Give it an antihistamine (Benadryl). See chart on page 73 for dosage.
- If you know that your pet has had serious allergic reactions to insect stings or spider bites, ask a vet to prescribe epinephrine[2] (or another medication) in the form of a pen injector, for use in case of emergency. You should keep one in your first-aid kit and take one with you when you're exercising outdoors with your pet.
- Stay with the animal for a few hours if it's had a vaccination. If a reaction occurs, administer first aid before visiting a vet.

---

2. Epinephrine is another name for adrenaline, a hormone used to increase the heart rate, blood pressure, etc.

## Bites

All animals, whether wild or domestic, bite to defend themselves. That's why domestic animals are particularly susceptible to this type of injury. It's important, therefore, to know how to deal with bites because they often carry – and can sometimes transmit – contagious and fatal diseases, like rabies.

Tomcats and unneutered dogs often fight with other males in order to stake out their territories and attract females in heat. This generally explains the bites that you might see on your pet. On the other hand, an animal that roams far afield is more likely to run into, and be attacked by, wild animals.

| CAUSES | SYMPTOMS |
|---|---|
| • Fights.<br>• Wild-animal attacks. | • A bite wound usually leaves two deep teeth marks in the skin and muscle.<br>• Abrasions to the skin; sensitive when touched.<br>• Swelling.<br>• Bleeding.<br>• Abscess develops after a few days. You'll notice swelling around the wound and the presence of pus. The site is red and painful. The abscess may burst, producing a foul smell.<br>• Loss of appetite.<br>• Fever, above 39.4° C (103° F).<br>• Lethargy. |

**First aid**

- If fresh, clean the wound with tepid water and disinfect with iodine.
- Consult a vet. Animals, especially cats, have abundant bacterial flora in their mouths, making a bite wound a breeding ground for local and systemic infections.
- If an abscess appears, see a vet.
- If the abscess bursts, clean the wound with tepid water and apply iodine (wear latex gloves), then consult a vet.
- If your pet was bitten by a wild animal that later died, place the carcass in a sealed plastic bag (wear latex gloves) and take it to the vet. If the wild animal is alive, don't try to capture it, but report its whereabouts to your local wildlife officer.

## Snakebite

If you live in a snake-infested area, whether the snakes are venomous or not, don't let your pet roam freely. Keep your dog on a leash whenever you walk in the woods.

Before traveling abroad with your animal companion, inquire about local snakes. Not all snakes are venomous, however, but even the nonpoisonous kind is almost always painful and can cause infection.

**Non-venomous snakes**

Symptoms

A non-venomous snakebite leaves horseshoe-shaped teeth marks. It may sometimes resemble a superficial scratch and may or may not show teeth marks. Such bites are not dangerous and won't cause poisoning. But swelling and inflammation will follow, even if the wound is superficial.

**First aid**
- Shave the hair around the wound.
- Cleanse the wound with water and soap or an antiseptic solution, such as iodized soap.
- Apply a topical antibiotic ointment (Polysporin). Snakes have abundant bacterial flora in their mouths, and their bites are therefore a breeding ground for infection.
- In case of persistent bleeding, apply a dry sterile bandage.
- Monitor your pet for at least three hours following the snakebite. If swelling increases or pus is present, see a vet.

**Venomous snakes**

The most common venomous species in North America belong to the *Crotalidae* family, indigenous to the United States. Better known as pit vipers, they include the copperhead snake, the cottonmouth water moccasin, and a number of rattlesnake species. The coral snake, found in the American south and in Mexico, belongs to a different family, the *Elapidae*.

The pit viper has a triangular head, with a deep pit between eyes and nostrils. Its pupils are elliptical and it has a pair of fangs, used for injecting venom. How a snakebite affects a pet depends on the snake's size, the type and quantity of venom that has entered the bloodstream (neurotoxin, hemotoxin or a combination of both).

If snakebite is suspected, administer first aid and consult a vet immediately. A venomous snakebite will cause blood to gush from the wound, followed by swelling and pain, then by systemic and neurological symptoms. Left untreated, snakebite can lead to death.

| BITE SYMPTOMS | POISONING SYMPTOMS |
|---|---|
| • Bleeding or blood gushing from the wound.<br>• Change in behavior.<br>• Horseshoe-shaped bite wound, topped with two fang marks.<br>• Swelling.<br>• Breathing difficulty. | • Collapse.<br>• Convulsions.<br>• Diarrhea.<br>• Excessive salivation.<br>• Lethargy.<br>• Muscular spasms.<br>• Nausea and vomiting.<br>• Panting.<br>• Paralysis in affected area.<br>• Shock.<br>• Tissue death around the bite.<br>• Weakness. |

**First aid**
- Keep the animal calm. If overexcited, its heart rate will accelerate, causing the venom to spread more rapidly throughout the body.
- Remove the animal's collar to avoid strangulation (a serious allergic reaction may cause the neck to swell).
- Immobilize the animal. Hold it gently in your arms. If the animal is too heavy, lay it on a blanket or a board, to be carried by two people. Don't let the animal walk; doing so will accelerate the blood circulation and cause the venom to spread. If you're alone, walk slowly with the animal until you are out of the snake's range, then lay the animal down and administer first aid.
- If the bite is on a leg, lower the leg below the heart. (If you raise it, circulation will accelerate, carrying venom to the heart.)
- Wash the wound with soapy water.
- If possible, immobilize the affected leg with a compressive bandage (see page 108). The bandage should be just tight enough to immobilize the leg and slow down lymphatic and venous – but not arterial – circulation. Make sure you can still slip two fingers under the bandage. Do not remove the bandage before

arriving at the vet's office. On the other hand, do not leave the bandage in place for more than two hours. If you have a magazine or a newspaper, you can roll it around the affected leg to immobilize it.

- If the neck, face or legs swell, administer the antihistamine Benadryl (diphenhydramine): see Allergic Reactions, page 71.
- If necessary, administer CPR (see page 41) and artificial respiration (see page 34).
- Take the animal to the vet within four hours of the incident. The animal must be hospitalized and will need monitoring for at least eight hours, so as to make sure that all the toxins are completely eliminated from the system. As well, a venom antidote might have to be administered by a veterinarian.

---

**WHAT *NOT* TO DO IF YOUR PET SUFFERS SNAKEBITE**

- Don't apply ice to the wound to relieve pain. This will cause tissue death around the wound.
- Don't open the wound or try to suck out the venom.
- Don't apply a tourniquet. The animal could lose its leg.
- If you suspect a snakebite, don't wait for serious symptoms to appear before calling a vet. It sometimes takes three to four hours for symptoms to occur and by then it may be too late to act. If the animal has no immediate neurological symptoms, take care of the wound and consult a vet within four hours of the incident.

---

## Burns

Most burns can be avoided by observing simple safety measures, such as keeping your pet out of the kitchen when you prepare meals, checking the water temperature before bathing your cat, covering household electrical wires if your dog tends to chew on them, etc.

## Benign burns

Minor burns are not life-threatening, but painful nonetheless.

| CAUSES | SYMPTOMS |
|---|---|
| • Abrasive burns caused by an accident (a fall, being hit by a car, etc.).<br>• Contact with hot food, plate, furnace, heating pad.<br>• Electrical wires causing burns to the mouth and internal organs.<br>• Fire.<br>• Hot bathwater.<br>• Sunburn (radiation): snout, eyes. | • Blisters.<br>• Pain.<br>• Red and inflamed skin. |

### First aid

- Apply cold compresses over and around the burned area to reduce inflammation, pain and discomfort:
  - A gel pack is easy to manipulate and won't get the animal wet.
  - A bag of frozen, uncooked rice is ideal for emergencies, because it's flexible and fits snugly around the limbs.
  - Frozen aloe vera gel is also ideal for emergencies, excellent for treating minor burns.
- Do not use oily products (no butter). The body's healing mechanisms will regenerate superficial tissues.

### Severe burns

Second and third-degree burns cause serious damage both to superficial tissues and the deeper layers of the skin. They can be fatal and should be treated immediately. Provide first aid, then consult a vet as soon as possible.

| CAUSES | SYMPTOMS |
|---|---|
| • Abrasive burns as a result of an accident (a fall, being hit by a car).<br>• Electrical burns to mouth and internal organs (see page 83).<br>• Contact with hot food, plate, furnace, heating pad, etc.<br>• Hot bathwater.<br>• Sun exposure (radiation): snout, eyes.<br>• Fire. | • Animal refuses to move because of pain.<br>• Edema (caused by tissue damage and fluid loss in burned tissues).<br>• Shedding of burned skin.<br>• Weakness followed by shock. |

### First aid

- Calm the animal as you administer first aid. Keep it warm in case it is in shock.
- Cover the animal to prevent it from biting the damaged skin (animals tends to do so when in pain).
- Apply cold compresses – or a cold gel pack – to reduce pain and swelling.
- In the case of severe burns, the badly damaged skin leaves the animal vulnerable to local and systemic infections. Apply a clean dressing – a large piece of sterile gauze found in a first-aid kit, for example – to prevent contamination and infection from outside sources.
- If the first-aid kit includes a physiological solution or water, dampen the sterile gauze before applying it to the wound.

- Secure the dressing with a light bandage (adhesive cotton), making sure it's not too tight. A tight bandage will prevent blood flow to the injured tissues.
- Do not apply an oily ointment or cream on an open wound. The product will become encrusted in the burned skin and aggravate the wound.
- Check the animal's vital signs: heartbeat, respiratory rate, gum color.
- Be prepared to treat the animal for shock, even on your way to the vet.

> Second-degree burns are serious and require a vet's care
> as soon as possible.

## Chemical burns

Several household products contain chemicals that risk causing serious burns either to the skin or the digestive tube. To prevent accidents, store them away from animals.

| CAUSES | SYMPTOMS |
|---|---|
| • Acids.<br>• Bleach.<br>• Toxic agents apt to cause chemical burns.<br>• Petroleum by-products (gas and oil, for example).<br>• Household cleaners.<br>• Anti-flea insecticide: repeated use may cause skin irritation and burns, and eventually lesions to the central nervous system. If the animal develops a reaction to anti-flea products, treat it the way you would a burn.<br>• Hair dye. | • Fur discoloration.<br>• Itching.<br>• Red skin and swelling.<br>• Skin peeled off as a result of contact with acid. |

**First aid**

- If you suspect that the animal has been exposed to a chemical irritant (as listed above), rinse it with warm water for 15-30 minutes. But beware, some products are activated on contact with water, so call the poison-control center or a veterinarian if you don't know the nature of the chemical involved.
- If you're certain that the animal has either oil or gas on its coat or plantar (toe) pads, rub the affected area with a small amount of vegetable oil, then rinse off with dish detergent. If you give the animal a bath, do not add soap or moisturizer. This may cause the chemical to penetrate the skin or become encrusted in the hair.
- Discolored fur signals that the animal has been exposed to a chemical product. If the animal has long hair, shave off the affected part.
- The animal will tend to lick itself as it tries to get rid of the chemical irritant. It goes without saying that ingesting these products will worsen its condition. (See Chapter 4, page 57).
- If the chemical has entered the eye, rinse it with cold running water for a few minutes; if the chemical is a powder, blow it off or remove it with a hairdryer, and rinse the eye with running water. Then call a vet immediately. An eye injury is always an emergency.
- First aid should give the animal some relief, but if it still exhibits discomfort, has red spots or itchy skin or eyes, take the animal to the vet. And don't forget to bring the guilty container.

**Electrical burns**

Kittens and puppies are more prone to electrical burns than adult animals, because they are curious and tend to chew on anything they can find. However, simple safety measures will prevent most of these accidents.

| CAUSE | SYMPTOMS |
|---|---|
| • Electrical wiring within reach of an animal. | • Animal unconscious with a piece of electrical wire in its mouth or a wire nearby.<br>• A conscious animal that has been electrocuted may show burn wounds a few days after the incident. The animal may go into hiding, moan, slobber (saliva sometimes tinged with blood), or bring its legs to its snout (sign of pain caused by ulcers).<br>• Bad breath (possibly caused by burns to the tongue or lips).<br>• Loss of appetite due to pain. |

**First aid**
- If you find your pet with an electrical wire in its mouth or nearby, cut the power and unplug the wire.
- Check for vital signs and administer CPR, if necessary.
- Treat the animal for shock, if necessary.
- Take the animal to the vet (electrical burns may damage internal organs).

## Choking or Respiratory Obstruction

Choking occurs when an animal's breathing passages are blocked or the trachea is compressed.

| CAUSES | SYMPTOMS |
|---|---|
| • Allergy or anaphylactic reaction to medication, insect bites and stings, or vaccination, causing neck and throat to swell and animal to choke.<br>• Inflammation and bleeding caused by trauma or accident.<br>• Respiratory infections potentially leading to pulmonary bleeding.<br>• Small toys, bone or food lodged in throat.<br>• Trauma to nasal, pharynx, larynx or trachea passages after a fall or other accident.<br>• Tumors inside and around throat causing coughing fits and breathing difficulty. | • An animal normally breathes between coughing fits. If you're not sure if your pet is coughing or choking, treat it for choking. Coughing can lead to choking.<br>• Bluish gums, sign that oxygen fails to get to tissue. Animal chokes.<br>• Choking may lead to loss of consciousness and respiratory arrest.<br>• Retching and breathing difficulty. |

**First aid**

*If the animal is conscious:*

- Keep an animal as calm as possible if it chokes or has a coughing fit. Let it cough and expectorate, if necessary.
- Don't strike the animal on the head or chest. It will panic and the swallowed object will remain stuck.
- Poke a finger into the mouth, toward the middle of the throat and at the base of the tongue. If you see the obstruction and can remove it without agitating the animal, then proceed.

- Remove all vomit or secretions in the trachea.
- Be cautious: an agitated animal can bite as a reflex.
- Make sure you don't pull the "Adam's apple" by mistake (see page 33).

*If the animal is unconscious:*
- Try to clear the breathing passages with your finger. Pull the tongue to one side and inspect the mouth and throat to locate the obstruction.
- Check to see if the animal is breathing. If not, blow into its snout twice to ventilate. If the chest doesn't rise, something is obstructing the trachea. Remove the obstruction with your finger.
- Hold the animal head down. If it is small, hold it by the hips and shake it gently and rhythmically. If it's a large dog, hold its hind legs, as you would a wheelbarrow, head down and resting on the front legs. If the obstruction doesn't come out, perform the Heimlich maneuver (see page 42).
- The animal may suffer cardiac arrest after breathing stops. Clear the air passages and make sure that air enters the lungs before performing CPR. It's useless to massage the heart if air can't enter the lungs.
- If the heart stops, perform artificial respiration combined with chest compressions (external heart massage): two insufflations for every 12 compressions (see page 41).
- If you're alone, provide emergency care on the spot (Heimlich maneuver and CPR), rather than taking the animal to a vet.
- If there are two of you, one person can begin and continue CPR while the other drives to the veterinary clinic.
- It's important to have your choking animal examined by a vet afterward. For one thing, the obstruction may have caused lesions to the air passages. For another, in a panic or for lack of experience, you may have injured the animal when performing CPR or the Heimlich maneuver.

# Constipation

Constipation is the retention of stools for longer than 24 hours.

| Causes | Symptoms |
|---|---|
| • Abscess in the anal region.<br>• Dirty litter box.<br>• Dry-food diet.<br>• Fiber-poor diet.<br>• Hairball.<br>• Inactivity.<br>• Ingestion of a foreign object.<br>• Insufficient water intake.<br>• Liver, kidney or thyroid disease.<br>• Spinal injury.<br>• Stress.<br>• Tumors. | • No trace of stools for more than two days.<br>• Small, hard stools.<br>• Animal moaning and straining while in the litter box.<br>• Occasional loss of appetite.<br>• Vomiting due to evacuation efforts. |

**First aid**

- If the animal excretes small, hard stools, supplement its diet with pumpkin-pie filling, Metamucil, or prune juice: 5 to 10 ml (1 to 2 teaspoons) for a cat, and 10 to 20 ml (2 to 4 teaspoons) for a dog.
- If the animal doesn't defecate for more than a day, see a vet. The problem may be more serious than you think.
- If the animal had no bowel movements for more than three days, it may have developed a condition called megacolon, which requires extraction of the stools manually or by surgery. See a vet immediately.
- If the animal is regularly constipated, it should be thoroughly examined by a vet. It may suffer from an unrelated illness.

## Diarrhea

Diarrhea is characterized by the increased frequency or watery flow of stools. The seriousness of the condition varies according to the presence of toxins. All cases of diarrhea must be treated, because it may indicate, among other things, that the animal has ingested a toxic or otherwise irritating substance.

The intestine is lined with a special mucus, made up of so-called villus cells, which aid the absorption of nutriments during digestion. Whenever these cells are damaged or destroyed, they can no longer absorb nutriments, nor retain water, leading to an increasingly liquid diarrhea.

| Causes | Symptoms |
| --- | --- |
| <ul><li>Allergies (food or preservatives).</li><li>Glandular illness (thyroid).</li><li>Drug therapy (prescribed or over the counter).</li><li>Imbalance and destruction of the gastrointestinal mucous membrane by toxins, poison, bacteria or viruses.</li><li>Internal parasites.</li><li>Medications (anti-inflammatory drugs, aspirin).</li><li>Metabolic illness (liver, pancreas).</li><li>Poisoning.</li><li>Stress.</li><li>Tumors in digestive system or other organs.</li></ul> | <ul><li>Frequent trips outside.</li><li>Soft or liquid stools.</li><li>Mucus in the stools.</li><li>Blood in the stools.</li><li>Moaning.</li><li>Weakness.</li><li>Dehydration (see page 18).</li></ul> |

### First aid
An animal suffering from diarrhea for more than a day will become dehydrated and require professional care.

- If you suspect that the diarrhea has been caused by ingesting poison or ran-cid food, administer first aid for food poisoning (see page 57) and consult a vet.
- If the diarrhea is linked to a change in the animal's diet and it is otherwise in good health, replace the new food — and substitute small amounts of chicken or boiled ground beef and cooked white rice, for a day or two. If the diarrhea is controlled following this treatment, gradually restore the animal's normal food. You can also provide some yogurt daily, so as to restore its intestinal bac-terial flora: 5 ml (1 teaspoon) for a cat, and 5-10 ml (1-2 teaspoons) for a dog, once or several times a day.
- If the diarrhea persists, even on a diet of boiled beef and rice, see a vet.
- If the animal is not vomiting, offer some water, but in small amounts. That will help prevent dehydration due to water loss through the stools. You can pro-vide a solution rich in electrolytes (in your first-aid kit or by using Gatorade mixed with a little water) in order to replace the missing electrolytes.
- An animal suffering from diarrhea should never be deprived of water, unless it vomits.
- If the animal doesn't vomit but is too weak to drink, give it an ice cube to lick, on the way to the vet.
- If the animal suffers from frequent diarrhea, with mucus or blood present, and seems weak or depressed, if it vomits or won't eat, see a vet immediately.
- If an animal is less than a year or older than 10 and suffers from diarrhea, con-sult a vet without delay, for such animals are more fragile and their physical condition can deteriorate rapidly.

## Dislocations

Whenever a bone is disconnected from the joint, it is called a dislocation. The knees and hips are most frequently affected.

| CAUSES | SYMPTOMS |
|---|---|
| • Hip dysplasia (a genetic problem).<br>• Ligament weakness resulting in dislocation of the hip or knee joints.<br>• Trauma caused by a fall or vehicle collision. | • Animal moves on only three legs.<br>• Limping.<br>• Joint pain, especially when the limb is moving.<br>• Abnormal position of the paw in relation to the joint: the paw appears twisted or hangs loosely.<br>• Swelling around the dislocated joint.<br>• The affected limb seems shorter. |

**First aid**
- Check vital signs; apply CPR if required (see page 41).
- Check for signs of shock (see page 38).
- Keep the animal calm.
- Muzzle the animal.
- If necessary, control bleeding by applying a compressive bandage (see page 108).
- Handle the animal carefully so as to avoid moving the joint.
- Take the animal to the vet. Do not let it walk.

## Drowning

Drowning claims many domestic animals every year. Dogs and cats are instinctive swimmers, but there are situations where even their natural skills are unavailing.

Basic safety rules are therefore in order. Keep a constant eye on your pet if it jumps into a lake or pool. Also look out for cramps and exhaustion. We've all heard stories of pets drowning because they couldn't climb out of a swimming pool, so make sure that your own pool is properly gated.

As they say, an ounce of prevention is worth a pound of cure. Why not give your pet a lifejacket, adapted to its weight and size, whenever you're both near the water?

### First aid

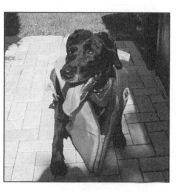

- **Small dog or cat**: Hold the animal by its hind legs, head down, and gently shake it in order to expel the water from its lungs and snout.
- **Medium-size or large animal**: Lift its hind legs and let the animal stand on its forelegs. Keep the hind legs elevated until all water has left its lungs.
- Lay the animal on its side so that the head is lower than the body (it helps to place a blanket under the rump) so that water in the lungs can run out.
- Check vital signs and perform CPR, if necessary (see page 41).
- If air doesn't enter the lungs, repeat steps 1 and 2; then perform CPR again.
- Wrap the animal in a blanket to keep it warm.
- Consult a vet as soon as possible. Continue CPR on the way to the vet, if necessary.

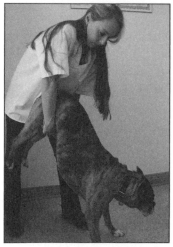

## Ecchymosis (Bruising)

When a blood vessel ruptures, the blood spreads through the subcutaneous tissue and forms red, blue and yellow spots on the skin. These are ecchymoses, or bruises, more familiarly.

| CAUSES | SYMPTOMS |
|---|---|
| • Blood disorder.<br>• Poisoning (rat poison).<br>• Trauma (blow, fall, pinching, animal bite). | • Swelling.<br>• Skin marbled with blue or yellow.<br>• Visible red spots in places where the fur is sparse.<br>• Local hematoma at site of wound, caused by the accumulation of blood flowing from the injured blood vessels.<br>• Painful to the touch. |

### First aid
- Apply cold compresses for 15 minutes three or four times a day until the swelling subsides.
- If ecchymoses appear or the body is covered with spots, consult a vet (chance of poisoning).
- If the swelling does not subside after 24 hours, consult a vet (there may be a fracture).

## Epilepsy and Convulsions

Epilepsy is a neurological illness characterized by sudden convulsions and loss of consciousness. A seizure occurs when neurons in the cerebral cortex fire up in an uncontrollable but synchronized way, rather like small electrical shocks occurring in a specific part of the brain — a reaction that will never occur under normal conditions. Epilepsy can be partial if it only affects certain parts of the cerebral cortex, or generalized if it affects the entire brain.

When an animal suffers repeated convulsive episodes, it is referred to as being epileptic. Hereditary factors seem to play a role in triggering seizures, among other causes. A brief convulsion usually lasts from 30 seconds to a few minutes and won't be harmful. However, repeated and prolonged convulsions are extremely dangerous.

| CAUSES | SYMPTOMS |
|---|---|
| • Cardiovascular disorder.<br>• Infection, fever.<br>• Metabolic illness (liver or kidneys).<br>• Muscular and skeletal dysfunction.<br>• Neurological dysfunction.<br>• Poisoning (lead, antifreeze, insecticides, rat poison).<br>• Trauma.<br>• Tumors. | **Before convulsions**<br>• An animal may sense the onset of convulsions and generally show early warning signs.<br>• Unusual behavior; animal seems lost or upset.<br>• Excessive lip licking.<br>• Muscle contractions of face and body.<br><br>**During convulsions**<br>• Gradual loss of consciousness (leading to fainting).<br>• Involuntary movement of the limbs: lying on its side, the animal beats the air with its legs as if running.<br>• Contraction of the skin muscles.<br>• Trembling.<br>• Excessive salivation.<br>• Involuntary urination and defecation. |

| Causes | Symptoms (cont'd.) |
|---|---|
| | **After convulsions**<br>• Disorientation or confusion.<br>• Unusual behavior that may last for 24 hours; animal's personality, gait and mind are affected.<br>• Headaches: animal presses its head against a wall. |

**First aid**

- Let the convulsions follow their course, as it is impossible to suppress them.
- Keep the animal in a quiet environment.
- Remove any nearby objects to prevent injury.
- Lay the animal on the ground so it won't fall down.
- Be gentle, as rough handling can prolong convulsions.
- As soon as the animal returns to normal, calm and reassure it.
- Subdue lighting and reduce noise levels, so as to avoid prolonging the seizure.
- Consult a vet after the animal has recovered.
- Epilepsy is not an illness in itself, but is provoked by another medical problem. That's why it's important to consult a vet if the animal is subject to convulsive episodes.

## Eye Injuries

Eye injuries often consist of lacerations to the eyelids or eyeball. What's more, bruises sustained from a blow or a fall may cause swelling or bleeding in the head or around the eyes. The pet is likely to rub its eyes and the lids may swell or bleed.

## Conjunctivitis

Conjunctivitis is the inflammation of the mucous membrane lining the inner surface of the eyelids.

| CAUSES | SYMPTOMS |
|---|---|
| • Allergies.<br>• Chemical irritants.<br>• Foreign objects.<br>• Infections, either bacterial, viral or fungal. | • Edema and reddening of the lower eyelid.<br>• Itchy eyes, causing edema to the eyelids (allergies).<br>• Pain.<br>• Scratching the eyes (due to itching or pain).<br>• Watering (pus). |

### First aid
- Gently apply cold compresses or ice, which help reduce pain and swelling.
- Keep the eye clean (clean off the pus) and rinse with water.
- Apply an antibiotic ointment to the eyes (first-aid kit).
- See a vet.

## Eyeball injuries

The most common cause of trauma is the presence of a foreign object in the eye. Another condition, though much rarer, is eyeball protuberance, or proptosis – that is, when the eyeball pops out of the socket.

### Foreign objects

Some foreign objects are large enough to be visible on the eyeball or eyelid. Others are too small to detect or are embedded underneath the eyelids; but they can still scratch or even lacerate the surface of the cornea and damage the eye.

| Causes | Symptoms |
|---|---|
| • Chemical irritants (see Chemical burns, page 87). <br> • Presence of particles in the eye: wood, metal (dust), plastic, rocks, etc. | • Bleeding. <br> • Scratching of eyes. <br> • Squinting. <br> • Swollen eyelids. <br> • Visible foreign object in the eye. |

### First aid

- If the foreign object is invisible, rinse the eye with cold water to flush out the particle.
- Apply cold compresses to relieve swelling and pain, making sure not to put pressure on the eye. You can also use a damp towel or a cold gel pack.

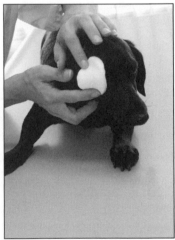

- Even if the foreign object is visible – a twig, for example – do not try to remove it. You'll risk damaging the eye and causing internal bleeding.
- Prevent the animal from scratching or rubbing its eyes. Apply a damp gauze compress to protect the injured eye, topping it with a cardboard, plastic or polystyrene cup (a yogurt container will also do). Cover the healthy eye as well, with a light, dry gauze pad. In this way, the animal can't make eye movements and risk aggravating the injury.
- Secure the dressings with a bandage, making sure not to put pressure on the eyes.

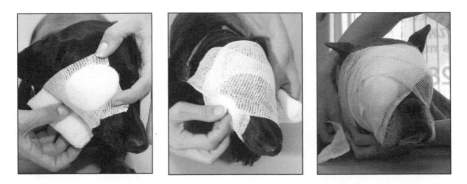

- Place an Elizabethan collar around the animal's neck to prevent it from touching the eye. If the collar is unavailable, you can make one from a cardboard box and adhesive tape. Cut a large round section, making a hole in the middle the size of the animal's neck. The cone must be 12.5 to 25 cm (5-10 in.) from the tip of the snout.
- See a vet immediately.

## Eyeball protuberance

Fortunately, eyeball protuberance or proptosis (eyeball popped from its socket) occurs only rarely, affecting mostly flat-snouted dogs and cats (Pekinese, Shih Tzu, bulldogs, Persians, etc.). It does need immediate attention, but deal with it calmly.

| CAUSES | SYMPTOMS |
| --- | --- |
| • Fight with another animal.<br>• Head trauma (blow, collision, fall, etc.).<br>• Strangulation by a leash. | • Eyeball hanging outside the socket, with closed eyelids behind it.<br>• Swollen eyeball. |

**First aid**
- Calm the animal.
- Do not try to replace the eyeball, you'll risk aggravating the injury and destroying the eye.
- Keep the eye moist by applying several layers of sterile gauze soaked in cold water. Place a cup or container over the dressing to prevent accidental pressure. Wrap a bandage around the head to keep everything in place.
- See a vet immediately.

## Foreign Objects

Frequently, a foreign object will penetrate an animal's body (legs, eyes or elsewhere). Note that an encounter with a porcupine generally leaves visible and painful traces on your pet. The presence of a foreign object requires immediate intervention, because infection commonly results.

### Foreign objects beneath the skin's surface
A free-ranging animal will walk on all manner of debris such as broken glass, metal or wood fragments, etc. It may also run into wild animals.

| Causes | Symptoms |
|---|---|
| • Metal fragments.<br>• Encounter with a porcupine. | • Swelling around the wound.<br>• If a foreign object (splinter, glass, metal) has penetrated a plantar pad, the animal hesitates to walk on the affected leg.<br>• Pain and sensitivity to the touch.<br>• Constant licking of the affected area.<br>• Porcupine bristles on the snout or elsewhere on animal's body. |

**First aid**

*If porcupine bristles are planted in the skin, proceed as follows:*
- Cut the ends of the bristles with scissors in order to squeeze the air from inside the bristles. The dog will feel better when you remove them.
- Grasp each bristle with tweezers and pull with a brisk movement.
- Disinfect the wound with an iodine solution.
- If the animal is restless and refuses to be treated, do not insist. Take it to the vet. Your pet may need a sedative.

*If the foreign object is a visible wood or metal splinter, proceed as follows:*
- Disinfect the forceps with rubbing alcohol and use them to remove the splinter.
- If the splinter is just beneath the skin, scrape it off with a disinfected needle, then remove the object with forceps.

*If the foreign object is a piece of glass:*
Remove it only if it's large enough to be grasped with forceps, making sure not to aggravate the cut. Do not try to remove small, unretrievable pieces. Soak the leg in warm water and Epsom salts (or sea salt) for 10 minutes. This will help the wound get rid of any glass dust that might have accumulated.
- After the object is removed, clean and soak the affected limb in a mixture of warm water and Epsom salts (or sea salt) for 10-15 minutes per day, so as to reduce swelling, until complete recovery.
- If the wound won't heal properly or the animal shows signs of discomfort, see a vet. The wound may be deeper than it appears and tiny pieces of debris are perhaps still present.

## Foreign objects deeply embedded in the skin

| CAUSES | SYMPTOM |
|---|---|
| • Walk in the woods (twigs stuck in the skin).<br>• Fights with other dogs.<br>• A fall on something hard (stick, small sharp object). | • Visible foreign object. |

### First aid
- Calm and immobilize the animal.
- Check for vital signs. Administer CPR if necessary (see page 41).
- Check to see whether the animal is in a state of shock, and treat it accordingly (see page 38).

- If the wound is bleeding, control it by applying direct pressure. Make sure not to remove the foreign object so as not to cause additional bleeding (see page 107).
- Immobilize the foreign object. Wrap gauze or a clean cloth (first-aid kit) around the object to prevent it from moving. For better results, use adhesive tape or another piece of cotton that you can wrap around the body or the limb. Make sure you don't apply too much pressure on the wound or abdomen.
- Don't try to remove the foreign object, because you risk causing or aggravating the bleeding and damaging the subcutaneous tissues.
- See a vet immediately. Transport the animal with great care and don't allow it to walk. Use a box if the animal is small, or a flat board if it's large. Immobilize the animal during the trip to the vet.

## Fractures

A bone fracture is often the result of a trauma, or collision with a vehicle, a fall, or caused by a falling object.

| CAUSES | SYMPTOMS |
|---|---|
| <ul><li>Accidents.</li><li>Aging.</li><li>Bone condition.</li><li>Malnutrition.</li><li>Vigorous games.</li></ul> | <ul><li>The most visible symptom is an abnormal position or movement of a limb. A fractured toe is enough to cause an animal to limp.</li><li>Pain in or near the fracture between two joints. The animal will moan if the spot is touched.</li><li>Swelling and hematoma.</li></ul> |

**First aid**
- Handle the animal carefully, a fracture is very painful and improper handling can damage the surrounding tissues.
- If a dog is injured, muzzle it.
- Cats should be wrapped in a blanket as they can also bite.
- If necessary, control bleeding by applying a compressive bandage (see page 108).

## Applying a splint

A splint is used to immobilize the affected limb and prevent aggravation of the injury, until the animal can receive veterinary care.

### Foreleg splint

- Any material sufficiently strong and stiff will serve as a splint.
- You can use two pieces of wood or cardboard placed lengthwise along the injured leg; or magazines or newspapers rolled around the leg and held in place with adhesive tape.

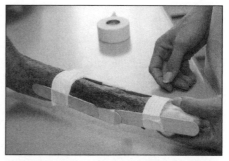

- You can also use a towel to immobilize the fractured limb. Pass the towel underneath the limb and roll it up in such a way that it forms a tight fit on either side of the limb, then keep it in place with adhesive tape.
- Position the splint so that it will immobilize the joints above and below the fracture and wrap the

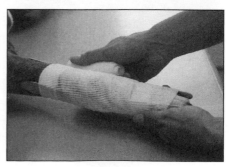

splint and the limb with adhesive tape to keep it secure. Next, wrap the limb with conforming bandage (gauze), then cover the whole thing with an elastic cohesive bandage to keep the dressing in place.

• A splint must never be overly tight!

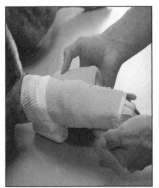

*Hind leg splint*
• Wrap the leg from toes to thigh in several layers of cotton bandage roll (in the first-aid kit). The cotton provides a thick surface, yet not too dense, which will help reduce the swelling and protect the leg.
• Keep the cotton bandage in place with adhesive tape or an elastic cohesive bandage. If no bandage material is available, use the other leg for support and tie the two legs together.

## Open fracture

An open fracture is indicated when the bone protrudes through the skin at the injury site. In such cases, there is danger of bone and systemic infection.

| Causes | Symptoms |
|---|---|
| • Bad fall.<br>• Hit by an automobile.<br>• Rough-and-tumble games or trauma. | • An open fracture occurs when a bone pierces the skin.<br>• Severe pain.<br>• Moaning. |

**First aid**
- If the wound is not bleeding, rinse it with lukewarm salt water: 5 ml (1 teaspoon) of salt per liter of water.
- Place a clean compress on the wound (see page 108).
- See a vet immediately, whether or not the wound is bleeding.
- Do not attempt to reposition a bone that has broken through the skin.

## Frostbite

An animal's body possesses defense mechanisms against the cold, but if exposed to below-freezing temperatures for any length of time, the same mechanisms that preserve body heat and keep the animal alive can also produce a contrary effect, causing necrosis of the extremities: tips of the ears, tail, plantar pads and legs. This is called frostbite.

When a dog or cat is exposed to excessively cold temperatures, its body reacts in three stages:

1. The animal's fur acts as a protective cover like human skin: once in contact with the cold, it stands up. At that point, like the rest of us, the animal gets "goose bumps." The upright hair creates a small cushion of air which, warmed up by body heat, acts as an extra layer of insulation.
2. When body temperature drops, an involuntary reflex of the skeleton muscles — known as shivering — kicks in to generate heat. Human beings display the same reaction.
3. When exposed to temperatures below the freezing point, an animal is at risk. Its body reacts by contracting the peripheral blood vessels (vasoconstriction). This indicates that the body is sending blood to those organs that play a key role in keeping the animal alive. The blood then circulates throughout the body and, by means of vasoconstriction, the blood vessels located at the extremities shut down temporarily until body temperature returns to normal. At that point, if the animal cannot restore body heat or hasn't received first aid, it will suffer from frostbite. The affected tissues will be destroyed. Cats and dogs are often frostbitten on the tips of the ears, tail, plantar pads and, in males, the testicles.

| CAUSE | SYMPTOMS |
|---|---|
| • Prolonged exposure to below-freezing temperatures. | • Animal feels cold and shivers.<br>• Skin is bright red, then turns pale (vasoconstriction) and, finally, black (necrosis or tissue death). |

**First aid**
- Do not rub or massage the frozen tissues.
- Do not apply ice or snow.
- Do not submerge the animal in a bath, because its body temperature will drop, risking hypothermia (see page 121).
- Quickly warm up the affected area using tepid water and towels.
- If the frostbite is limited to a single leg or a paw, soak the frozen area only in a tub of tepid water, then gently dry after it has warmed up.
- Prevent the animal from mutilating itself. When the tissues are warm again, the animal will experience some discomfort and pain and will try to bite the affected area. The same thing will happen if the tissues are destroyed (necrotic).
- Wrap the animal in a blanket to keep warm (see page 122) and prevent self-injury.
- Take its temperature and check for signs of hyperthermia (excessive warming can overheat the animal). Administer appropriate first aid (see page 118).
- Consult a vet.

## Gastric Dilation

Gastric dilation, a condition affecting larger dogs in particular, is an abnormal bloating of the stomach, caused by the absorption of large amounts of air. The stomach inflates like a balloon and can rotate on itself, causing what is known as gastric torsion. The torsion puts pressure on the diaphragm, makes breathing difficult and compresses the main blood vessels located behind the heart (posterior to the vena cava), preventing the blood from returning to the heart. Gastric dilation demands urgent treatment, because the animal may die. See a vet as soon as possible.

| CAUSES | SYMPTOMS |
|---|---|
| • Eating too quickly.<br>• Ingesting large quantities of food and water.<br>• Vigorous exercise immediately before or after eating. | Symptoms appear a few hours after eating:<br>• Excessive salivation that causes the animal to slobber.<br>• Discomfort or restlessness: the animal moves around ceaselessly.<br>• Swollen abdomen (the stomach area resembles a balloon).<br>• Attempts to vomit (unable to do so owing to gastric torsion).<br>• Breathing difficulty.<br>• Blue-colored gums.<br>• Shock. |

**First aid**
- Check vital signs; apply cardiopulmonary resuscitation (CPR) if necessary (see page 41).
- Check to see if the animal is in a state of shock and administer first aid as needed (see page 38).

- Take the animal to a vet immediately. Massage it gently on the way. Apply no pressure to the abdomen.
- Use the same transportation technique as you would for an animal suffering from a spinal-column injury. Let the animal walk it if can, but go slowly, and don't hurry it along.

## Hemorrhage

Hemorrhage, or bleeding, is caused by a ruptured blood vessel owing to trauma. It may be external or internal. If external, there may be multiple causes: a cut on the plantar pad, a leg or some other part of the body. If internal, it could be due to organ damage (liver, kidneys, etc.). Blood loss of as little as 10 ml (two teaspoons) per kilogram (2.2 pounds) can send the pet into shock, not to mention heavy bleeding, which reduces blood flow and leads to shock even more rapidly, causing hypoxia – a condition of lowered oxygen levels in the blood. Hypoxia causes cell and tissue death in the blood-deprived area.

### External hemorrhage

No matter what kind of external bleeding occurs, it's important that you try to stop it immediately. Make sure that your first-aid kit contains the necessary material: gauze, cotton bandage roll, elastic bandages, adhesive bandages, scissors (see page 141).

| Causes | Symptoms |
|---|---|
| • Cuts.<br>• Lacerations. | • Bright red blood that spurts out rhythmically indicates an arterial hemorrhage, the most serious kind.<br>• Dark red blood that flows freely, without spurting, comes from a vein and is less serious than an arterial hemorrhage.<br>• Blood that oozes from a wound comes from the capillaries and is not considered serious. |

**First aid**

*Applying pressure to the wound*

Applying direct pressure to the wound often stops the hemorrhaging effectively. You need only place a clean cloth or gauze on the wound and apply steady pressure with fingers and hands. If cloth or gauze is unavailable, press straight down with your hand.

Do not remove the cloth or gauze even if it is blood-soaked. Simply add more layers and maintain pressure. This will help the blood coagulate.

Do not touch blood clots that have formed.

*Compressive bandage*

Once you've covered the wound with a clean cloth or gauze, top it off with a compressive bandage and apply pressure, using a cotton or gauze bandage roll.

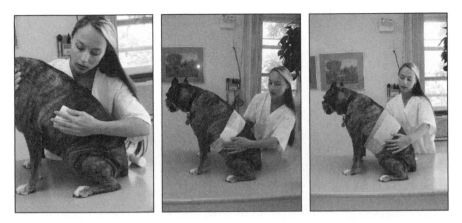

Keep the compressive bandage in place with an elastic tubular bandage (Co-Flex). It must not be too tight in order to avoid damaging the surrounding tissues or restricting circulation.

Use the commercial 3-M elastic bandage only if you're familiar with it, because it tends to cut off circulation. Elastic bandages provided in first-aid kits, such as Co-Flex, are quite safe.

### Elevation

If bleeding persists, even after you've applied a compressive bandage, elevate the affected limb or paw so the wound is above heart level. Blood pressure in the injured part is thus lowered, reducing the bleeding. Continue applying direct pressure on the elevated wound, adding compresses if necessary. Do not remove or change the first bandages that you've placed on the wound, you'll risk removing the blood clots that have formed in the meantime, and the wound will bleed again.

### Compressing the blood vessel in the injured limb

If bleeding still persists, even after you've elevated the wound, apply direct pressure on the vessel that supplies blood to the wounded limb.

- To control arterial bleeding, apply pressure with your hands between the wound and the location of the heart.
- To control venous bleeding, apply pressure below the wound.
- If a hind leg bleeds copiously, press a finger or thumb on the femoral artery, located in the groin area.
- If a foreleg bleeds, press a finger or thumb on the brachial artery, located on the inside of the leg.
- If the tail bleeds, press a finger at its base.

### Tourniquet method

A tourniquet is used to tighten a bandage so as to compress the arteries of a limb. This method is not risk-free, so employ it only if the bleeding is massive and therefore life-threatening. Always try to apply a compressive bandage or direct pressure on the wound first. If a tourniquet is essential, you'll know when to use it! But remember that it's only a temporary solution.

### Applying a tourniquet

- Use a necktie, belt or a 5-cm (2-in.) piece of fabric to make a tourniquet.
- Wrap the tourniquet twice around the limb, above the wound. Do not make a knot.
- Tighten gradually to reduce or stop the bleeding, but leave enough space for a finger to slip between limb and tourniquet.
- Bleeding should stop once you've pulled the two ends of the tourniquet around the limb. Make a compressive bandage.
- If bleeding has stopped, remove the tourniquet completely. Continue applying direct pressure as needed.
- Note the time at which you installed the tourniquet. After 5 to 10 minutes, slowly release the tourniquet. Do not leave it on for more than 10 minutes.

If bleeding persists, even after you've wrapped the two ends around the limb twice, proceed as follows:

- Place a short stick or similar implement (a "popsicle" stick or a branch) alongside the limb and secure it with a piece of fabric.
- Turn the stick to tighten the tourniquet until bleeding stops.
- Secure the newly positioned stick with another piece of fabric.
- Write down the time and stick the note on the bandage.
- Slowly release the tourniquet every 10 minutes for a 60-second interval, in order to permit normal blood flow to the injured limb.
- If bleeding stops after the tourniquet has been released, remove it completely.
- If the animal has lost a lot of blood, it may be in a state of shock. Control the bleeding first, then treat the animal for shock (see page 38).

---

If you leave the tourniquet in place for too long, it may cause tissue death and even the loss of the injured limb.

---

You've saved your pet's life by responding quickly with appropriate first-aid techniques. But hemorrhaging is a serious condition and the next step is to take the animal to a vet. Injuries involving wounds often cause substantial blood loss and systemic infections, which require surgery and sutures.

## Internal hemorrhage

Internal bleeding is harder to detect. An animal that's had a bad fall or been hit by a car may appear unharmed because it can walk, has no visible injuries and behaves normally. An owner, too, may think that the pet is simply a little shaken by the experience.

The animal may be too frightened to feel pain, or realize what has happened. Its "normal" behavior may be a symptom of the first stage of shock, and for all we know, the pet may even be suffering from internal hemorrhaging and its life may be in danger.

| CAUSES | SYMPTOMS |
|---|---|
| • Car accident (ruptured organs, such as the bladder).<br>• Gunshot wound.<br>• Illness.<br>• Poisoning (rat poison).<br>• Trauma (fall, collision, etc.). | • Cold extremities (tail, paws and ears). When there is blood loss, the body reacts by shutting off the blood flow (vasoconstriction) to the non-vital areas of the body so that the blood is diverted to the vital organs. This is why the extremities are cold.<br>• Pale-colored gums (check to see if the gums and the inside of eyelids are pale pink or white. They should be bright red).<br>• Slow capillary refill time. Press the gums with your finger: their color should go from white to red in less than three seconds. A longer duration suggests blood loss or a second stage of shock.<br>• The animal is highly agitated (tendency to run away when frightened) or unusually apathetic (first stage of shock).<br>• Bleeding from ears or nose (see pages 113-115).<br>• Blood in urine or stools, even if accident occurred a few days prior.<br>• Long intervals between breaths: the animal inhales deeply each time.<br>• Swollen abdomen, which may lead to shock (see page 38). |

**First aid**

If the animal displays one of the above symptoms, comfort it and call a vet at once.

Do not put pressure on the animal's abdomen as you transport it to the vet. This might rupture an already injured organ and cause massive bleeding. (See Transporting an Injured Animal, page 28.)

**Nosebleed**

A nosebleed can usually be dealt with easily, requiring basic first aid. But if bleeding persists, the blood may get sucked into the respiratory track. If blood loss is significant, the animal can experience a state of shock.

| CAUSES | SYMPTOM |
|---|---|
| • Coagulation problems. <br> • Ingestion of rat poison (Warfarin). <br> • Nasal tumors or ulcers. <br> • Snout trauma or injury. <br> • Vigorous and prolonged exercise. <br> • Violent sneezing. | • Bleeding from the snout. |

**First aid**

- The animal must stay calm: speak to it quietly and avoid restraining it. If an animal feels restricted or is forcibly held back, it will panic and bleeding will persist, preventing blood clots from forming. Apply ice cubes and gently elevate the snout. This will help blood clots to form.
- If the animal bleeds from the snout following a trauma (fall, traffic accident), it may go into shock and lose consciousness. See page 38 for shock treatment.
- Consult a vet as soon as bleeding is controlled, regardless of cause.

**Blood in the urine**
This condition requires a vet's care.

| CAUSES | SYMPTOMS |
|---|---|
| • Bacterial, fungal or viral infection.<br>• Bleeding (genetic condition or poisoning).<br>• Inflammation due to infection (presence of stones).<br>• Prostate disease.<br>• Renal infection.<br>• Trauma (ruptured bladder).<br>• Tumors.<br>• Urinary blockage (male cats). | • Traces of blood in urine.<br>• Blood in stools.<br>• Frequent expulsion of small quantities of urine and blood.<br>• Presence of blood on the fur of the genital area.<br>• Moaning while urinating. |

**First aid**
- If the animal eats and drinks normally and appears in good health, but traces of blood in the urine persist, the animal is probably suffering from a chronic health problem. Consult a vet for a complete examination.
- If the blood in the urine is dark red and there is more blood than urine, see a vet immediately.
- If small drops of blood are visible but the animal cannot urinate, see a vet immediately. It is an emergency (see Urinary Blockage, page 134).

## Bleeding on the surface of the ear

Animals that suffer from itchy ears, usually caused by mites, will scratch until their ears bleed. This is not an emergency, but you should still see a vet, because the situation may cause lesions in the ear canal. If you detect blood on the surface of, or inside, the ear, administer first aid as quickly as possible.

| CAUSES | SYMPTOMS |
|---|---|
| • Fight with another animal, causing ear lacerations.<br>• Hematoma on the ear: a ruptured blood vessel, for example, resulting from head blows or constant scratching (especially cats).<br>• Self-mutilation.<br>• Trauma: road accident, fall, etc. | • Thick ear (accumulated blood).<br>• Swollen, red ears.<br>• Bleeding from the ear. |

**First aid**

- If the ear surface bleeds, apply pressure with a clean cloth until bleeding stops.
- If bleeding persists, wrap a bandage around the head.
- Place a gauze compress on the wound, then wrap the ear from tip to base. If the dog's ears are set straight up, the injured ear should stay as is. On the other hand, if the ears are long and droopy, then lay the injured ear on the animal's neck.
- Wrap the gauze bandage two or three times around the animal's head and jaws. Secure the bandage with an elastic cohesive bandage.
- Make sure the bandage is not too tight, especially around the jaws, so the animal can continue to breathe freely. You should be able to easily slip two fingers under the bandage. If not, the bandage is too tight.
- See a vet.

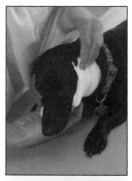

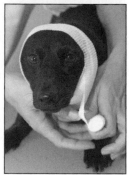

## Hyperglycemia

Hyperglycemia refers to above-normal levels of blood sugar, a condition that especially affects diabetic animals. Diabetes is a metabolic problem that causes an abnormal increase of blood sugar owing to insufficient insulin production. Like humans, diabetic animals need regular intakes of insulin, which can be administered either orally or by injection. Insulin dosage varies from animal to animal.

Incorrectly administered insulin may cause hyperglycemia. This condition must be treated immediately, because it can lead to coma and death.

| CAUSES | SYMPTOMS |
|---|---|
| • Incorrect insulin dose. A diabetic pet requires regular visits to the veterinary clinic so its insulin needs can be monitored properly. They fluctuate over time.<br>• Incorrectly administered insulin and irregular meal times.<br>• Other factors unrelated to diabetes may also bring on hyperglycemia, such as stress, or illnesses linked to the thyroid, liver, kidneys, etc. | • Vomiting, before and after meals.<br>• Breath and urine smelling of sugar.<br>• Loss of appetite.<br>• Dehydration. Animal eliminates more water than it drinks, owing to high blood sugar.<br>• Weakness.<br>• Increased respiratory rate (see Normal Respiratory Rates, page 13).<br>• Change in behavior (tendency to hide).<br>• State of shock. |

**First aid**
- Check vital signs and perform CPR if necessary (see page 41).
- Check to see if the animal is in a state of shock (see page 38).
- Hyperglycemia in a diabetic animal is an emergency. Consult a vet immediately. Take some insulin with you, in the case the vet doesn't have any on reserve.

## Hyperthermia

Hyperthermia, or heatstroke, occurs when body temperature is above normal, in other words, a fever resulting from exposure to intense heat and humidity. An animal will try to cool down by panting, a mechanism that helps reduce body heat. But if the pet is enclosed – inside a vehicle for example – panting will have the contrary effect, filling the ambient air with steam, thereby increasing heat and humidity further.

If body temperature exceeds 41.5 – 42.5°C (106.7 – 108.5°F), cellular functions are seriously affected, potentially leading to loss of consciousness, even death.

| CAUSES | SYMPTOMS |
|---|---|
| • Animal left inside a locked vehicle, either in direct sun or hot weather. This is a potentially deadly situation, even with a slightly open window.<br>• Animal left outside in hot, humid weather without water or shade.<br>• Certain short-snouted breeds – Shih Tzu, boxer, Pekinese, bulldog and Persian cat – are particularly sensitive to hyperthermia, because their flat faces make breathing difficult.<br>• Difficulty in adjusting to weather changes; very young or very old animals are particularly sensitive to excessive heat. | • Plantar pads perspiring.<br>• Breathing difficulty.<br>• Blood-streaked diarrhea.<br>• Accelerated respiratory and cardiac rates (see Vital Signs, pages 13 and 15).<br>• Panting.<br>• Salivation.<br>• Vomiting.<br>• Elevated body temperature (above 40°C or 104°F).<br>• Bright red mucus membranes.<br>• Short capillary refill time (less than a second).<br>• Dehydration.<br>• Apathy, lethargy (symptoms of intoxication).<br>• Shock. |

| Causes | Symptoms (cont'd.) |
|---|---|
| • Health problems: If a pet has epilepsy, heart or lung problems, it should never be exposed to excessively hot, humid weather.<br>• Intense exercise in hot, humid weather, even when the animal has plenty of water at its disposal.<br>• Thick-coated dogs (husky, German shepherd, Chow Chow). | • Epileptic seizure, collapse or coma. |

**First aid**
- The aim is to cool down the animal as quickly as possible, so that the body temperature can return to normal.
- If the pet is outside or in a car, lay it down in a cool, shady place.
- Check vital signs. Perform CPR (see page 41) and treat the animal for shock (see page 38), if necessary.
- Wet the animal with cold water. If you are at home, place the animal in the bathtub and turn on the cold shower.
- Soak towels – or anything you can find – in cold water and apply them to its head, neck, paws, chest and abdomen.
- Take the animal straight to the vet. Turn your car air conditioner up to maximum for the entire trip. If the animal is in shock, one person can perform CPR while the other drives.
- Apply rubbing alcohol on the plantar pads. This will cool down the animal.
- Continue the cooling process, taking the animal's body temperature every five minutes until you arrive at the vet's. Even after it has returned to normal (38.5 to 39.5°C, or 101.3 to 103.1°F), continue monitoring it to make sure that hypothermia won't set in (see page 121).

First aid is crucial in treating heatstroke. But your pet must be thoroughly examined by a vet soon after in order to avoid further complications, which can occur hours or even days later: kidney failure, for example, or problems with the digestive, neurological and cardiorespiratory systems.

## Hypoglycemia

Hypoglycemia refers to abnormally low blood-sugar levels, causing an animal's energy level to drop. While it mainly affects diabetic animals, hypoglycemia may also be caused by other medical problems. It is a serious condition and, if left untreated, can result in coma and death.

| CAUSES | SYMPTOMS |
|---|---|
| • Infection and tumors.<br>• Loss of appetite resulting from an illness, boredom when alone, a physical or emotional trauma.<br>• Vomiting following an insulin injection (diabetic animals).<br>• Weakness. | • Wobbly gait.<br>• Disorientation.<br>• Trembling.<br>• Epilepsy.<br>• Loss of consciousness. |

**First aid**
- Spread corn syrup on the gums (do not forcibly introduce it into the mouth). If it is unavailable, use sugar diluted in water, honey or sweet syrup (never chocolate). The aim is to give the animal glucose. Proceed even if the animal is unconscious.
- After administering corn syrup, take the animal to the vet.
- If the animal is not diabetic but exhibits any of the above symptoms, give it syrup all the same, and take it to the vet immediately.
- Check vital signs and perform CPR if necessary.

# Hypothermia

Hypothermia refers to below-normal body temperature, a condition that may cause shock, loss of consciousness, even death. Animals left outside in below-freezing temperatures are at risk of hypothermia. If your pet is frostbitten, for example, check for hypothermia. However, frostbite is by no means the only symptom: animals may very well suffer from hypothermia without being frostbitten.

| CAUSES | SYMPTOMS |
| --- | --- |
| • Animal is left outside, in below-freezing temperatures.<br>• Infection.<br>• Metabolic dysfunction. | • Below-normal body temperature (under 37.5°C or 99.5°F). Take rectal temperature (see page 12).<br>• Shivering (physiological reflex for countering the cold and keeping warm).<br>• Weak pulse. You should feel a strong, rhythmic beat by placing your index finger on the pet's femoral artery, located in the groin area. A slow, faint beat indicates poor circulation.<br>• If you're unable to take the animal's femoral pulse, focus on other symptoms.<br>• Weakness.<br>• Loss of consciousness.<br>• Shock (see page 38). |

**First aid**

- Cover the animal with a blanket to keep it warm.
- A hairdryer is a handy way to supply heat while another person prepares hot-water bottles and other heat-generating items.
- Heat a gel pack (or a small bag of uncooked rice) in a microwave oven for two, three minutes, then wrap in a towel to avoid burns.
- You can also use a heating pad, but don't place the animal on it directly. Cover it with a towel first. A weakened animal can't move and may get badly burned.
- Take the animal's rectal temperature every 10 to 15 minutes. Normal body temperature is between 38.5 and 39.1°C (101.3 – 102.3°F).
- Treat the animal for shock, if necessary (see page 38).
- Hypothermia is a life-threatening condition. So take the animal to a vet for a thorough examination once you've done whatever is necessary to keep it warm.
- When body temperature returns to normal, cease all warming operations. Excessive heat is also harmful (see Hyperthermia, page 118).

## Ingestion of a Pointed or Sharp Object

An animal may accidentally swallow glass ornaments, staples or other sharp or pointed objects. These may cause internal bleeding and damage the gastrointestinal tract.

**First aid**

- Soak cotton balls (natural, not the synthetic kind) in frozen coffee cream and feed them to your pet. The balls will wrap themselves around the cutting or pointed object in the digestive tube, preventing lesions and cuts to the fragile tissues.

- For a cat or small dog: give two cotton balls cut into small pieces.
- For a dog between 4.5 and 22.5 kilograms (10 to 50 pounds), give three to five whole cotton balls. The animal will swallow them with pleasure, considering them as treats.
- Check the animal's stools for the next few days. They will have odd shapes, which is normal. If you see traces of blood, consult a vet.
- Cotton is not harmful to animals, because it contains a natural protein, similar to that found in cat or dog hair.

## Injuries to Paws, Toes and Plantar Pads

An animal's feet are the most sensitive parts of its anatomy. The plantar pads resemble sponges and contain numerous blood vessels. As a result, they tend to bleed profusely after an injury, and take a long time to heal.

| CAUSES | SYMPTOMS |
|---|---|
| <ul><li>Burns and irritation caused by winter road salt.</li><li>Claws broken or torn.</li><li>Cut caused by ice, broken glass, foreign objects.</li><li>Fractures.</li><li>Frostbitten toes.</li><li>Perforation by a piece of wood, foreign object, a nail.</li><li>Cracked plantar pads due to the cold weather.</li></ul> | <ul><li>Bleeding from a cut or perforation.</li><li>Constant licking of the affected leg.</li><li>Limping.</li></ul> |

**First aid**

- Stop the bleeding. Apply a special powder to the wound (first-aid kit) or use cornstarch and a compressive bandage (see page 108).
- Rub cracked pads with petroleum gel (Vaseline) or an ointment laced with Vitamin E. Make the animal wear boots.
- To treat burns caused by road salt, rub the pads with an aloe gel or a homeoplasmine cream (see Homeopathic Products, p.154) and make the animal wear boots.
- For burns caused by cold weather, see Frostbite, page 104.
- Consult a vet once you've applied a bandage to the affected plantar pads. Do not remove the bandage in case bleeding reoccurs. Plantar pads are sensitive and may need a few stitches.

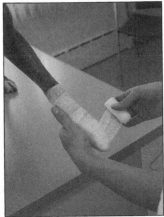

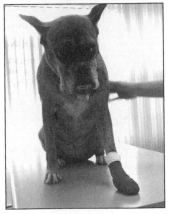

## Injured nails

Most nail injuries are minor and will heal quickly after first aid has been administered. However, in a day or two, check to see if your pet still limps, has a tendency to lick its wounds, or if the affected toe – and all the remaining toes for that matter – has swollen or reddened. If one of these symptoms persists, see your vet.

| CAUSES | SYMPTOMS |
|---|---|
| • Nails cut too short.<br>• Nails broken or torn following a fight or car accident.<br>• Cracked or shedding nails (medical condition). | • Bleeding toes.<br>• Limping.<br>• Constant licking of the affected leg.<br>• Moaning (small breeds in particular). |

**First aid**

- When bleeding occurs, press the injured area with a piece of gauze or a clean cloth.
- Use cornstarch or flour. Another alternative is to embed the affected nail in a clean bar of soap or in some paraffin.
- If you have a medication to prevent bleeding such as silver nitrate (available at pet shops), apply it immediately while maintaining the pressure for a few minutes. But use it only as a last resort because it can cause pain or a burning sensation, not to mention burns to the skin or eyes.
- If the paw continues to bleed, apply a compressive bandage (see page 108) and see a vet.

# Paraphimosis

Paraphimosis occurs when an animal's foreskin is pulled back and is caught behind the penis' head, causing swelling and blocking blood flow.

| CAUSES | SYMPTOMS |
|---|---|
| • Abnormal prepuce preventing foreskin's retraction.<br>• After mating, penis fails to retract into foreskin.<br>• Penis swollen due to infection. Erection occurs while dog licks itself, and swelling prevents foreskin's retraction.<br>• Prolonged erection, preventing foreskin from retracting to normal position.<br>• Swelling caused by frostbite. Penis freezes when dog urinates in snow or in below-freezing temperatures. | • Penis cannot retract into foreskin.<br>• Penis covered with dirt.<br>• Red, inflamed penis.<br>• Tip of penis black or blue (after being exposed for a long time). |

**First aid**
- Cleanse the penis gently with running water. If erect for some time, the penis will have dried up and be covered with dirt.
- Apply ice cubes if there's swelling.
- Lubricate the penis with gel (K-Y jelly) to keep it moist, so that it can eventually retract into the foreskin. If not, consult a veterinarian.

# Parasites

## External parasites

External parasites are blood-sucking bugs, such as fleas, mites and ticks, that either cling to an animal's fur or lodge deep within the skin folds.

Although external parasites don't require immediate treatment, you should still consult a vet. Some parasites cause an allergic reaction or cutaneous problems, while others can transmit potentially fatal diseases.

## Fleas

Fleas are hopping insects, a domestic animal's parasites. They can carry disease and even transmit internal parasites. A flea-infested pet doesn't necessarily scratch itself. Lesions are caused by the animal's allergy to bites.

## Checking for fleas

- Place the dog or cat on a white surface and shake the hair to shed the black-colored flea excrement. Wet the droppings: if they leave a red trace, you know that your pet has fleas.
- Fleas typically lodge between an animal's thighs, on the abdomen or around the neck.

If you do find fleas, don't panic. As long as your pet is around, the fleas will prefer to stay on them rather than jump on you. There are many effective anti-flea products on the market. Ask your vet for advice.

## Ticks

Ticks are blood-sucking parasites that cling to the skin of various domestic and wild animals. They can transmit different infectious diseases.

**Dislodging ticks**

- Wear latex gloves.
- Spray a small amount of anti-tick or anti-flea product on the insect. If an anti-flea spray is unavailable, apply rubbing alcohol, petroleum gel (Vaseline) or mineral oil, using a cotton ball or a Q-tip. The tick will emerge within 30 to 60 seconds.
- As soon as the tick's head emerges, grasp it with forceps.
- Wait until the head is completely exposed before pulling on it. The whole insect will thus be removed, eliminating all risk of infection.
- Don't use matchsticks to remove a tick. The pet may get burned!
- It's important to remove a tick before it has a chance to transmit diseases to cats, dogs and even humans. Place the insect in a container, adding some alcohol, and take it to a vet for identification.
- Apply an antibiotic ointment or rubbing alcohol on the bite.
- If the tick's head is still stuck in or beneath the skin (a black dot), remove it as you would a splinter, using forceps or a credit card. If you can't, see a vet.
- If the swelling or redness persists for more than two days, consult a vet.

> Your pet is susceptible to a number of external parasites.
> A veterinarian can tell you how to control them.

## Internal parasites

Internal parasites – such as the common roundworm, tapeworm and hookworm – live and feed inside the animal's digestive tube and other organs. Intestinal worms delay growth, causing lesions in the digestive system, even hypoglycemia in kittens and puppies. Several types are transmittable both to animals and humans. If the problem is untreated, it may even cause death.

| CAUSES | SYMPTOMS |
|---|---|
| • Tapeworms transmitted by mice that cats love to eat.<br>• Infested female transmitting parasites to fetuses through placenta or to newborn animals through mother's milk (roundworm, hookworm).<br>• Fleas carrying immature tapeworms that, if ingested by pet, will develop in its digestive tube.<br>• Pets that eat animal excrement (susceptible to roundworms, tapeworms or hookworms).<br>• Poor hygiene (pet-boarding facilities, grooming salons). | • Roundworm: resembling a piece of spaghetti. Found in animal stools or vomit.<br>• Tapeworm: resembling small rice grains in stools or around the anus.<br>• Hookworm: difficult to identify, but causes blood-streaked diarrhea. |

**Care**

- If you spot worms in your pet's stools or vomit, note their size, color and shape or take a sample to a vet (wear latex gloves). It's not an emergency, but you should still consult a vet as soon as possible.
- If your pet looks sick, won't eat, is dehydrated and weak, vomits, or has blood and worms in its stools, see a vet: it's an emergency.
- Ask for stool analysis when you take your pet for its annual checkup.

## Rectal prolapse

Rectal prolapse occurs when a full layer of rectal tissue slides through the anal orifice.

| CAUSE | SYMPTOMS |
|-------|----------|
| • Straining to defecate owing to constipation (kittens and puppies). | • A sausage-like reddish mass, large or small, protruding from anal orifice.<br>• Swelling.<br>• Necrosis (dark red or black tissues). |

**First aid**

- Clean the protruding tissue with cold or tepid water.
- Apply lubricant gel.
- Push the tissue back into the anus, gently but steadily.
- If it returns to its proper place, the animal will recover.
- If not, apply lubricant gel (K-Y jelly) with a gauze or cloth to keep the exposed tissues moist, thus avoiding necrosis.

## Scrapes

Scratches and abrasions on the skin's surface are fairly benign and usually don't require a veterinarian's attention.

| CAUSES | SYMPTOMS |
| --- | --- |
| • A wound (the animal slips on cement or asphalt after an accident).<br>• Rubbing its head or snout against the bars of a cage. | • Skin scratches.<br>• Clumps of hair torn out.<br>• Oozing of blood.<br>• Redness and inflammation. |

**First aid**
- Shave the hair around the wound.
- Wash the wound in tepid or cold running water, to get rid of dirt and debris (the bathtub is ideal). If need be, bottled water is a good way to clean the wound.
- Disinfect the wound with clean gauze and an iodine solution (in the first-aid kit).
- Apply a topical antibiotic cream (Polysporin or the equivalent, in the first-aid kit or available from the vet).
- If the pain and swelling last longer than 24 hours and there is a discharge of pus, the wound may be deeper. Consult a vet in order to prevent a systemic infection.

## Skunk Spray

Don't be alarmed if your pet comes home smelling like a skunk. To eliminate the foul odor, you need only rinse the animal with the following formula:

**First aid**
- If the animal was sprayed in the eyes and face, rinse thoroughly with cold water.
- Bathe the pet in water with the following ingredients:

| | |
|---|---|
| 1 liter (4 cups) | Hydrogen peroxide (3%) |
| 50 ml (¼ cup) | Baking soda (paste) |
| 5 ml (1 teaspoon) | Dish detergent |
| 5 to 10 ml (1 to 2 teaspoons) | Vanilla extract |

The detergent will isolate the chemical agent (butenyl) that produces the foul smell. It will in turn be neutralized by the reaction of the baking soda and hydrogen peroxide, while the vanilla extract will give the affected pet a pleasant scent.

## Sprains and Muscle Pulls

A sprain is a painful lesion caused by violent trauma to a joint, with or without tearing of ligaments. A strain is an excessive stretching of a muscle.

| CAUSES | SYMPTOMS |
|---|---|
| • Loss of balance or fall (long nails that get stuck in the carpet).<br>• Overexercise, especially in dogs.<br>• Weakness.<br>• Rough-and-tumble games. | • Swelling.<br>• Limping.<br>• Refusal to move.<br>• Pain (the animal moans and groans).<br>• Sensitive to the touch. |

**First aid**

- Apply cold compresses, or a cold gel pack, to the wounds.
- Keep the animal quiet, allowing it outside only to relieve itself.
- Restrain the animal from jumping up, exercising, going up the stairs. If you must limit its movements, keep it in a restricted area.
- If there is no improvement after 24 or 48 hours or the condition worsens, see a vet; it could be a broken bone.
- Consult a vet to see whether a painkiller is required.

## Trauma to the Spinal Column

Injuries to the spinal column are always serious, because of the inherent risk of neurological damage or broken vertebrae, which often have devastating consequences, such as paralysis. Fortunately, "serious" doesn't mean hopeless.

| CAUSES | SYMPTOMS |
|---|---|
| • Fall.<br>• In cats, hind leg paralysis (following a thrombosis).<br>• Miniature breeds (dachshund, for example) are more prone to back injuries (discal hernia).<br>• Nervous disorder.<br>• Traffic accident.<br>• Virus. | Symptoms vary according to injury's gravity and location on spinal column:<br>• Abnormal gait, stiff disposition.<br>• Bent spinal column.<br>• Dilated anal opening.<br>• No reaction to pain (when toes or legs are pinched, for example).<br>• Pain in neck and back.<br>• Paralyzed legs: limp or stiff muscles.<br>• Uncontrolled release of urine or stools.<br>• Weak legs: animal probably unable to support own weight. |

**First aid**
- Check vital signs and perform CPR if necessary (see page 41).
- Check to see if the animal is in shock (see page 38).
- Calm the animal.
- Avoid all spinal-column movements.
- Transport the animal to a vet on a rigid surface (see page 28) as soon as possible. The inflammation around the injury may compress and damage the nerves, further aggravating the situation.

## Urinary Blockage

Urinary blockage occurs when there is an obstruction in the urethra, the duct that carries urine from the bladder to the penis or vulva.

Urinary blockage affects all cats and dogs, but primarily male cats, because their narrow urethra tends to accumulate infected debris that will eventually prevent urine from flowing out of the bladder. While a female cat is less prone to this condition, she is still susceptible to infection.

Urinary blockage causes the bladder to bloat with urine, growing so hard that it can burst. The urea, a poisonous substance present in the urine, backs up into the kidneys and then the bloodstream, a situation that can cause death within 48 hours if untreated. It's imperative, therefore, that you consult a vet as soon as you suspect a blockage, because by that time the animal will have already suffered the toxic effects of a urinary blockage.

| CAUSES | SYMPTOMS |
|---|---|
| • Chronic bladder infection.<br>• Kidney disease.<br>• Kidney stones.<br>• Prostate problems.<br>• Tumors.<br>• Urinary mineral deposits (often associated with poor-quality food). | • Animal moans when it tries to urinate.<br>• Animal crouches to urinate, but only a few drops of urine or blood emerge.<br>• Cat trying to urinate in kitchen sink, bathtub – anywhere but the litter box.<br>• Frequent visits to the litter box.<br>• Prolonged stay in the litter box (as in cases of constipation).<br>• Dog asking frequently to be let out.<br>• Licking the genital region.<br>• Swelling in the genital region.<br>• Lack of appetite.<br>• Lethargy.<br>• Depression (the animal goes into hiding, looks for cool areas in the house).<br>• Heartbeat slowing down.<br>• Coma. |

**First aid**
- Urinary blockage is a medical emergency. Call the vet!
- During the trip to the vet, do not press on the abdomen because the bladder may burst.
- If the animal is small, take it in a box. Remove the lid, if there is one, so you can settle the animal in gently.

## Vomiting

Nausea and vomiting in dogs and cats can indicate metabolic problems as well as other conditions. Normally, vomiting is not cause for concern, but be vigilant nevertheless, and watch out for signs of dehydration, or any other disorder or trauma.

| CAUSES | SYMPTOMS |
|---|---|
| • Hairballs in stomach.<br>• Illness.<br>• Ingestion of grass or plants.<br>• Irritation in digestive tube.<br>• Poisoning.<br>• Presence of foreign object in stomach.<br>• Quick absorption of foods. | • Vomiting.<br>• Severe vomiting after eating. |

### First aid
- It's normal for cats to regurgitate hairballs from time to time, and it is painless. A laxative paste, available at a vet's office or specialty stores, will help the hairballs pass through the digestive tube and emerge with the stools.
- A healthy animal may often swallow grass or plants to induce vomiting, a natural mechanism for getting rid of bile. But make sure your pet doesn't ingest herbicide- or insecticide-treated grass or poisonous plants.
- If an animal eats too quickly, it may vomit as a nervous reflex. To help your pet slow down, feed it twice a day, offering little snacks between meals (carrots, apples, bananas, red peppers, etc.). For a miniature dog, place a tennis ball in its dish, and make it eat around the ball. But don't use this technique with large dogs – they may accidentally swallow the ball.

- If an animal exhibits signs of illness (apathy, diarrhea, fever, frequent vomiting, loss of appetite), take its food away, but continue offering it water as long as it can tolerate it. If not, apply honey to the gums in order to avoid hypoglycemia (see page 120) and consult a vet.
- If an animal vomits food and water, remove all food for 12 hours and consult a vet. Give the animal ice cubes in the meantime: if it has vomited, it may be dehydrated.
- If the animal vomits, but seems otherwise healthy (no signs of fever or weakness), give it an electrolyte solution in water (first-aid kit) or Gatorade as soon as it can drink without any nausea. Consult a vet.

## Wounds

Skin cuts and perforations can often occur: during walks in the woods, fishing trips, etc. They need immediate attention to avoid bleeding and risk of infection.

### Gunshot wounds
Hunting dogs and abused animals are the most common victims of gunshot wounds.

### First aid
- Calm the animal.
- Check for vital signs; administer CPR, if necessary (see page 41).
- Control bleeding with a compress (see page 108). If the bullet hole is visible, cover it with petroleum gel (Vaseline) and a bandage. Keep the dressing in place with whatever you have on hand, even a piece of clothing. Make sure the bandage is not so tight that it interferes with breathing.
- If the animal is in a state of shock, treat it accordingly (see page 38).
- Take the animal to the vet immediately, on a rigid surface if possible. Do not let the animal walk, even if it attempts to. This will aggravate bleeding and send the animal into shock.

## Lacerations

A laceration is a deep cut or tear in the skin.

| Causes | Symptoms |
|---|---|
| • Animal fights.<br>• Accident during grooming or nail clipping.<br>• Sharp object. | • Bleeding.<br>• Open wound (muscles, tendons, visible tendons).<br>• Skin cut, which may be deep and affect subcutaneous tissues, veins, arteries, ligaments, tendons, muscles and bones. |

### First aid

- If the cut is minor (light bleeding on skin surface), stop the bleeding and apply a dressing. Shave the hair around the wound, then clean and disinfect it. Apply a piece of sterile gauze with an antibiotic ointment. Cover the gauze with a conforming cotton bandage and wrap the limb. The bandage should be snug, but not too tight. Top it all off with an elastic cohesive bandage. Finally, apply an adhesive tape at each end of the bandage, one half on the dressing, the other on the hair.
- If the cut is deep and bleeds profusely (arterial hemorrhaging, for example), apply a compressive bandage (see page 108).

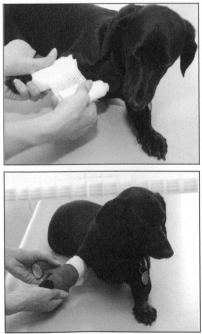

- Check for vital signs and shock symptoms, performing CPR if necessary (see Shock, page 38). As previously noted, bleeding may cause shock.
- Consult a vet: sutures may be required for deep cuts.

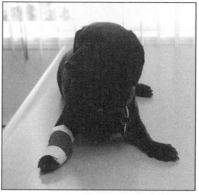

## Perforations

A perforation is a fairly deep hole in the skin caused by a sharp object – a fish hook, for example. Such accidents are generally avoidable. Also, don't forget basic safety rules.

| Cause | Symptoms |
|---|---|
| • Wound caused by a sharp object: nail, thumbtack, broken glass, fish hook, etc. | • Bleeding.<br>• Bruising.<br>• Deep wound, large or small.<br>• Painful to the touch.<br>• Swelling, redness, inflammation. |

**First aid**
- Control bleeding (see page 108).
- Check vital signs. Perform CPR if necessary (see page 41).
- If possible, shave the hair around the wound.
- Remove all visible material (claw, thumbtack, staple, piece of wood) as long as they are not too deeply embedded in the skin (see "Foreign Objects Deeply Embedded in the Skin," page 100).

- Clean the wound with tepid water, disinfect with iodine and apply an antibiotic ointment.
- Bandage the wound to keep it clean and avoid infection:
    - Apply sterile gauze and antibiotic ointment on the wound.
    - Secure the gauze by bandaging the limb snugly with the conforming bandage.
    - Top it all off with an elastic cohesive bandage. Always make sure the bandage is not too tight.
- Consult a vet.

**Fish hook**

A cat or dog playing near a fishing pole can easily get hurt on the face, lips, snout and legs with a fish hook. It may also swallow the object as it tries to get rid of it. The same accident can occur if a dog eats a dead fish with a hook still in its mouth.

**First aid**

Take the animal to a vet. If this is not possible, provide first aid as follows:
- Push the fish hook out of the wound so you can see the barb.
- Cut the barb with a pair of pliers.
- Pull the rest of the hook out through the point of entry.
- Clean the wound and disinfect with an iodine solution.
- Apply an antibiotic ointment to the wound.
- See a vet.
- If the hook is caught in your pet's mouth while it's still attached to the fishing pole, don't try to remove it. Don't feed the animal and seek veterinary care immediately.

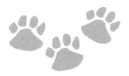

# ANNEX 1
# THE FIRST-AID KIT

**A** plastic box is all you need to house your first-aid kit. Keep it at home or in the car. Note important telephone numbers inside the lid: those of your veterinarian, the veterinary clinic's 24-hour service, the local poison-control center, and so on. When you're out walking your pet, take the kit with you, carrying it in a vinyl or waterproof bag attached to your belt.

Consult your vet, first-aid instructor, local pharmacist and CPR center about the kit's contents. Medication and disinfectants should carry expiry dates, and should be renewed or replaced accordingly. Check with your vet to make sure that there are no contra-indications — in other words, that your pet can safely use whatever medication is prescribed in an emergency, based on the animal's medical history.

## A first-aid kit should contain the following:

Adhesive tape
Antibacterial ointment (Hibitane, Polysporin or other), available at a vet's office or
    pharmacy
Antibacterial soap; Hibitane
Antihistamines, such as Benadryl (diphenhydramine, in correct dosages)
Antiseptic
Bandage scissors
Coated aspirin for relieving pain and reducing fever: FOR DOGS ONLY (see your
    vet for dosage directions)
Conforming bandage (cotton roll): 12.9-cm (2-in.) width
Corn starch (for treating bleeding nails)
Corn syrup (for treating hypoglycemia)
Disposable diapers or pads for compressing bandages (in case of bleeding)
Diarrhea medication; strawberry extract (5 ml or 1 teaspoon twice daily), or Pepto
    Bismol
Elastic cohesive bandage (Co-flex)
Emergency thermal blanket
Epinephrine or similar medication, such as cortisone, in pen-injector form
Epsom salts (for disinfecting wounds and reducing inflammation)
Eye lubricant
Forceps
Gel pack (or a small bag of uncooked rice)
Hydrogen peroxide (3%), to induce vomiting or for disinfecting wounds
Insulin (pen-injector form) for diabetic animals (prescribed by a vet)
Iodine (for disinfecting wounds)
Latex gloves
Nail clippers
Nylon leash
Old plastic credit cards for removing stings

Ophthalmic ointment; Polysporin
Paint-mixing sticks for making splints
Petroleum gel (Vaseline)
Q-tips
Sterile gauze pads (all sizes)
Sterile saline solution (for rinsing eyes and wounds)
Stethoscope
Syringes (25 cm$^3$), for cleaning wounds or giving water to sick pets
Table salt (to induce vomiting)
Thermometer (digital variety is more efficient than rectal)
Towel

Note: You can obtain a complete first-aid and CPR kit (for animals or humans) at any first-aid instructor's office. First-aid center for animals: www.kilookas.com

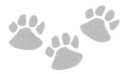

# ANNEX 2
# HOMEOPATHIC REMEDIES

**H**omeopathic remedies are safe, non-toxic and a helpful asset in an emergency. Don't hesitate to use them as you administer first aid to an animal in distress. They can help relieve discomfort and even improve the animal's general physical condition.

The remedies come in granule, pellet, liquid or cream form, and are also present in various solutions. For emergency situations, granules are more convenient to administer (dilutions appropriate for emergencies range from 5-7 CH with the exception of *Apis mellifica*, which should have a dilution of 7 CH or higher). Pellets are generally introduced directly into an animal's mouth. If the pet refuses to take them, dissolve the pellets in cold water and offer it as a drink, thereby sparing the animal added anxiety. The homeopathic remedy will be absorbed by the mucous membranes (tongue and gums). Cream is for external use. Make sure you clean the affected area before applying a thin layer of homeopathic cream, followed by a bandage, if necessary.

It is safe to administer several homeopathic remedies simultaneously, as they will not cause undesirable side effects. Homeopathic remedies are available at pharmacies, a holistic vet's office, or even from Internet companies, such as Kilookas (www.kilookas.com).

The following tables indicate the usage for various homeopathic products.

| SYMPTOMS | HOMEOPATHIC PRODUCTS |
|---|---|
| **Absence of lactation** | *Urtica urens* |
| **Allergy to insect bites and stings**<br>Itching | *Urtica urens*<br>*Hypericum perforatum*<br>*Ledum palustre* |
| Breathing difficulty | Poumon Histamine (Boiron) |
| Red and swollen skin | *Apis mellifica* |
| **Birthing difficulties** (all stages) | *Caulophyllum*<br>*Actaea racemosa* |
| **Bladder infection** (moaning during urination and presence of blood in urine) | *Cantharis vesicatoria*<br>*Aconitum napellus*<br>*Berberis vulgaris* |
| **Burns and scrapes** | *Cantharis vesicatoria*<br>*Apis mellifica*<br>Homeoplasmine cream (Boiron)<br>*Hypericum perforatum*<br>*Urtica urens* |
| **Car accident** | *Aconitum napellus*<br>*Arnica montana*<br>*Belladonna*<br>*Hamamelis*<br>*Apis mellifica* |

| SYMPTOMS | HOMEOPATHIC PRODUCTS |
| --- | --- |
| **Cold**<br>Sneezing with nose and eye secretions caused by infection (pus): begin with homeopathic treatment then consult a vet. | *Kalium bichromicum* |
| **Constipation** (small, hard stools) | *Nux vomica* |
| **Convulsions** | *Belladonna*<br>*Colubrina* |
| **Coughing** | Stodal syrup (Boiron)<br>Dogs: 1 teaspoon, 2-3 times daily<br>Cats: $^1/_2$ teaspoon, twice daily |
| **Diarrhea** | *Arsenicum album*<br>*Lipecachina* |
| **Diarrhea** (due to emotional shock) | *Staphysagria*<br>*Aconitum napellus* |
| **Diarrhea with flatulence** | *Licopodium clavatum* |
| **Ears** (red and swollen) | *Belladonna* |
| **Ecchymoses and sprains** | *Arnica montana*<br>*Apis mellifica*<br>*Hamamelis* |
| **Eye allergy**<br>Itchy eyes | *Urtica urens* |

| SYMPTOMS | HOMEOPATHIC PRODUCTS |
|---|---|
| Redness and irritation | Eye solution (Optalia by Boiron, for example): 2-3 times daily. Homeoplasmine cream (Boiron): apply a thin layer to eyelids and around eyes twice daily. |
| Eye secretions and swollen eyelids | *Arnica montana* <br> *Euphrasia officinalis* |
| **Eyes** <br> Cornea injury | *Ledum palustre* |
| Eyeball injury | *Symphytum officinale* |
| Conjunctivitis | *Euphrasia officinalis* <br> *Kalium bichromicum* <br> *Apis mellifica* |
| **Fractures** | *Arnica montana* <br> *Apis mellifica* <br> *Hamamelis* <br> *Symphytum* |
| **Frostbite** (pain) | *Aconitum napellus* <br> Homeoplasmine cream (Boiron) |
| **Gestation** (prevention) | *Calcarea phosphorica* <br> *Caulophyllum* <br> *Hypericum perforatum* |
| **Hairballs** | *Nux vomica* |

| SYMPTOMS | HOMEOPATHIC PRODUCTS |
|---|---|
| **Heatstroke** | *Glonoinum* <br> *Bryonia alba* <br> *Natrum muriaticum* <br> *Belladonna* |
| **Hemorrhage** | *Arnica montana* <br> *Erigeron* <br> *Hamamelis* (dark-colored venous blood) <br> *Millefolium* (red arterial blood) <br> *Aconitum napellus* (red arterial blood) <br> *Phosphorus* |
| **Injuries** <br> Tail or nails | *Hypericum* |
| To the head | *Arnica montana* <br> *Belladonna* <br> *Aconitum napellus* |
| To the vertebral (back) | *Hypericum perforatum* <br> *Bryonia alba* <br> *Arnica montana* |
| **Mammary glands: congested and hardened** <br> Intense pain: animal refuses to move | *Phytolacca decandra* MT <br><br> *Bryonia alba* |
| **Mastitis** (infection and swelling of the mammary glands) | |

| SYMPTOMS | HOMEOPATHIC PRODUCTS |
|---|---|
| Swelling | *Belladonna* |
| Infection | *Hepar sulphuris* |
| **Motion sickness** (nausea and profuse salivation) | *Petroleum* |
| **Paralysis** | *Aconitum napellus*<br>*Arnica montana*<br>*Belladonna*<br>*Hamamelis*<br>*Apis mellifica* |
| **Poisoning** | *Nux vomica* |
| **Recovering from surgery** | *Arnica montana*<br>*Staphysagria*<br>*Belladonna* |
| **Scrapes/Abrasions** | *Arnica montana*<br>*Hypericum perforatum*<br>*Calendula* topical lotion |
| **Shock** (panic state) | *Aconitum napellus*<br>*Arnica montana* |

| Symptoms | Homeopathic Products |
|---|---|
| **Sunburn** (redness, skin lesions) | *Cantharis vesicatoria*<br>*Apis mellifica*<br>*Urtica urens*<br>*Belladonna*<br>*Aconitum* |
| **Swollen tissues** | *Belladonna*<br>*Ferrum phosphoricum* |
| **Teething or toothache** | *Chamomillia* (drinkable ampoules) |
| **Urinary blockage** (inability to urinate, moaning) | *Sarsaparilla*<br>*Lycopodium clavatum*<br>*Berberis vulgaris* |
| **Weakness** | *Carbo vegetabilis* |
| **Wounds**<br>Gunshot wounds | *Ledum palustre*<br>*Belladonna*<br>*Apis mellifica* |
| Lacerations | *Staphysagria*<br>*Calendula* lotion<br>*Hypericum perforatum*<br>*Arnica montana*<br>*Apis mellifica* |

| HOMEOPATHIC PRODUCTS | INDICATIONS |
|---|---|
| *Actaea racemosa* | Weak and intermittent contractions during labor (three pellets every half-hour). |
| *Aconitum napellus* | Head injuries; shock; paralysis; frostbite; bleeding due to trauma; bladder infection. |
| *Apis mellifica* | Inflammation or edema (eyelids, skin, muscles); meningitis due to allergies and traumatic injuries. |
| *Arnica montana* | Trauma; lesions; stress; ecchymoses; fractures; sprains; muscle or ligament trauma; traumatic shock; post-surgery remedy. |
| *Arsenicum album* | Infection due to injury, skin irritation or food poisoning (diarrhea and vomiting). |
| *Belladonna* | Cutaneous congestion (redness); pain and sensation of heat (eyelids, abdomen, ears, plantar pads); heatstroke. |
| *Berberis vulgaris* | Symptoms of urinary infection: painful urination; presence of blood in urine. |
| *Bryonia alba* | Intense pain caused by congested and inflamed mammary glands; fever (heatstroke). |

| HOMEOPATHIC PRODUCTS | INDICATIONS |
|---|---|
| Carbo vegetabilis | Breathing difficulty. |
| Calcarea phosphorica | Helps gestating females and newborn animals to absorb calcium; prevents growth problems in newborn animals: three pellets weekly until weaning. |
| Calendula officinalis TM (Calendula topical lotion) | Open wounds and lesions (stimulates immune system). |
| Cantharis vesicatoria | Skin irritations and swelling due to burns: sunburns; helps relieve the burning sensation associated with bladder infections. |
| Caulophyllum | Helps to dilate the cervical canal during the first stage of labor: three pellets twice weekly during the last three weeks of gestation; during birth: three pellets every half-hour. |
| Chamomillia | Intense pain; light injury; toothache (kittens and puppies). |
| China rubra | Blood-tinged diarrhea due to food poisoning; abdomen sensitive to the touch; flatulence; fever. |
| Euphrasia officinalis | Clear nasal secretions (runny nose); swollen eyelids; red eyes; conjunctivitis — symptoms associated with allergies. Stimulates immune system. |

| HOMEOPATHIC PRODUCTS | INDICATIONS |
| --- | --- |
| Ferrum phosphoricum | Painful and swollen ears due to injury or frostbite. |
| Glonoinum | Congestion; violent headache; lack of coordination; lethargy; helps reduce cerebral edema. |
| Hamamelis | Bleeding (dark-colored venous blood); hematoma. |
| Homeoplasmine cream (Calendula officinalis MT, Phytolacca decandra MT, Bryonia dioica MT) | First-degree burns and frostbite. Reduces tissue redness and inflammation and accelerates the healing process. |
| Hypericum perforatum | Traumas to nerve endings; intense pain along the nerves or at their endings. |
| Ipecacuanha (Ipeca) | Nausea, vomiting due to food poisoning; diarrhea (with or without blood). |
| Kalium bichromicum | Respiratory infections (presence of pus in nose and eyes). |
| Ledum palustre | Skin eruptions and itching due to injuries; infected wounds caused by insect bites. Helps in the healing process |

| HOMEOPATHIC PRODUCTS | INDICATIONS |
|---|---|
| *Lycopodium clavatum* | Diarrhea with flatulence due to food poisoning. Helps prevent urinary blockage and recurrent urinary infections in cats. |
| *Natrum muriaticum* | Heatstroke. For preventive measures: five pellets twice daily prior to lengthy sun exposure. |
| *Nux vomica* | Food poisoning; vomiting; constipation; hairballs. |
| *Petroleum* | Motion sickness (nausea and vomiting during car rides). |
| *Phytolacca decandra* MT | Congested and tender mammary glands. |
| Poumon Histamine (Boiron) | Homeopathic antihistamine (helps to reduce pulmonary edema caused by severe allergic reaction). |
| *Sarsaparilla* | Helps to dissolve crystals and debris in the urethra (male cats, which are most susceptible to urinary blockage). |
| *Staphysagria* | Diarrhea caused by emotional shock; self-injuries (cuts, allergic itching). To be used after surgery; promotes scarring. |

| HOMEOPATHIC PRODUCTS | INDICATIONS |
|---|---|
| Stodal syrup | Coughing. |
| *Symphytum officinale* | Eyeball and bone traumas; pain. |
| *Urtica urens* | Itching and redness (eyelids, skin) due to allergies, first-degree burns and frostbite; also helps to reduce mammary congestion. |

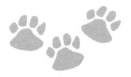

# REFERENCES

Bister and Kirk. *Handbook of Veterinary Procedures and Emergency Treatment,* Fourth Edition, U.S.A., W.B. Saunders Company, 1985.

Bonagura, John D. et al. *Kirk's Current Veterinary Therapy XII Small Animal Practice,* U.S.A., W.B. Saunders Company, 1995.

Cunningham, James G. *"Textbook of Veterinary Physiology,"* from *Thermoregulation,* Chapter 52, Second Edition, U.S.A., W.B. Saunders Company, 1997.

Ettinger, Stephen J. and C. Edward Feldman. *Textbook of Veterinary Internal Medicine,* Fourth Edition, Vol. 1, U.S.A., W.B. Saunders Company, 1995.

Fowler, Murray E. DVM. *Plant Poisoning in Small Companion Animals.* U.S.A., Ralston Purina Company, 1981.

Fraser, Clarence M. et al. *"The Merck Veterinary Manual,"* from *Toxicology,* Part VII, Sixth Edition, Rathway, U.S.A., Merck & Co. Inc., 1986.

Guermonprez, Michel et al. *Matière médicale homéopathique,* Third Edition, France, Boiron, 1989.

Guindon, Paul DMV. *Matière médicale homéopathique pour chiens et chats.* Montréal, Éditeur: Paul Guindon, 2000.

Osweiler, Gary D. *Toxicology. The National Veterinary Medical Series.* Williams and Wilkins Science Review, 1996.

Picard, Philippe. *Conseiller l'homéopathie.* France, Éditions Boiron, 1990.

Pratt, Paul W. *Medical Nursing for Animal Health Technicians*, First Edition, Goleta, CA., American Veterinary Publications Inc., 1985.

Schoen, Allen M. and Susan G. Wynn. *"Complementary and Alternative Veterinary Medicine. Principles and Practice,"* from *Veterinary Homeopathy Principles and Practice*, Chapter 26, St. Louis, MO, Mosby Inc., 1998.

Stein, Diane. *Natural Healing for Dogs and Cats*, pp. 105, 121. Freedom, CA, The Crossing Press, 1993.

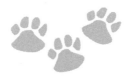

# ACKNOWLEDGMENTS

This book is dedicated to all animal lovers and to those who have made them part of their families.

A great deal of love and energy lies behind the making of this book every step of the way, and I want to thank everyone who helped me realize my objective. I drew personal inspiration from all the owners and their animal companions, and I thank them from the bottom of my heart.

Thank-you to my family whose constant support and encouragement have motivated me: to my mother, to Nadya and Pablo. Thanks also to my friends Diane and Tanya, and their dogs Buddy and Brandy. To Dr. Clayes, a veterinary acupuncturist, president of the Canadian Association of Veterinary Acupuncturists, for his advice, and to Dr. Guindon, a veterinarian who, from the outset, offered support and professional advice: my thanks and deepest gratitude.

Thank-you to the owners of Ali and Victor (Madame Philie and Dr. Guindon), who agreed to allow photos of their dogs to be used in the book.

And finally a special note of thanks to my publisher and his wonderful staff, as well as my photographer friends, Norm Edwards, Tanya Jocich and Tim Brien.

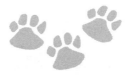

# CONTENTS

Printed in Canada
at Imprimeries Transcontinental Inc.
in September 2004.